CRITICAL ACCLAIM F

Perfection Sal

Delightful . . . There are two stories here, one about American cooking and one about American women.

—BARBARA EHRENREICH, *The New York Times Book Review*

A comprehensive, droll social history of a curious movement that's responsible for everything from nutritional education programs to TV dinners. —MAUREEN CORRIGAN, *The Village Voice*

Fascinating . . . a serious book, a must for the shelves of students of social, women's, and culinary history.

—MICHELE SLUNG, *New York Newsday*

Shapiro's very readable book helps explain why middle-class Americans developed a preference for a cuisine that sacrifices taste to the pure and the plastic.

—JOYCE S. TOOMRE, *Library Journal*

In this important book, Laura Shapiro traces the beginning of the domestic science movement and recounts its remarkable success in diverting the energies of vast numbers of women into docile acceptance of separate but equal status in those areas. The work is well researched and fascinating reading.

—KAREN HESS, *Ms.*

Laura Shapiro, a writer who knows how to charm as well as inform, has crammed the pages of her lively social history with anecdotal goodies and vivid portraits.

—LAURA MATHEWS, *Glamour*

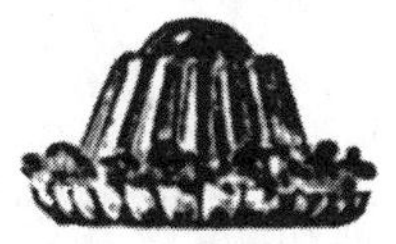

PERFECTION SALAD

Women and Cooking at the Turn of the Century

by

LAURA SHAPIRO

North Point Press
Farrar, Straus and Giroux
New York

*Published in Canada by HarperCollins*CanadaLtd
Printed in the United States of America
Designed by Cynthia Krupat
North Point Press edition, 1995

Library of Congress Cataloging-in-Publication Data
Shapiro, Laura.
Perfection salad.
Bibliography
Includes index.
1. Home economics—Study and teaching—United States—History. 2. Cookery—Study and teaching—United States—History. 3. Diet—United States—History. 4. Nutrition—Study and teaching—United States—History. I. Title.
TX173.S44 1986 641.5'0973 85-25402

Grateful acknowledgment is made to the following for their courtesy in granting access to their collections: The American Antiquarian Society, Worcester, Mass.: selections from the Lizzie A. Wilson Goodenough Diaries; The Colonel Miriam E. Perry Goll Archives at Simmons College, Boston, Mass.: selections from the minutes of the Boston Cooking School Committee; The Houghton Library, Harvard University: selections from the Marietta Greenough papers; The Massachusetts Historical Society, Boston, Mass.: selections from the letters of Ellen H. Richards and Edward Atkinson; Margo Miller: selections from the letters of Mrs. Dexter Perkins and Fannie Farmer; The Arthur and Elizabeth Schlesinger Library, Radcliffe College: selections from the papers of Christine Frederick, Edith Raymond, and the Mothers Club of Cambridge; The Sophia Smith Collection, Smith College: selections from the papers and letters of Ellen Richards.

For my parents

Contents

Perfection Salad

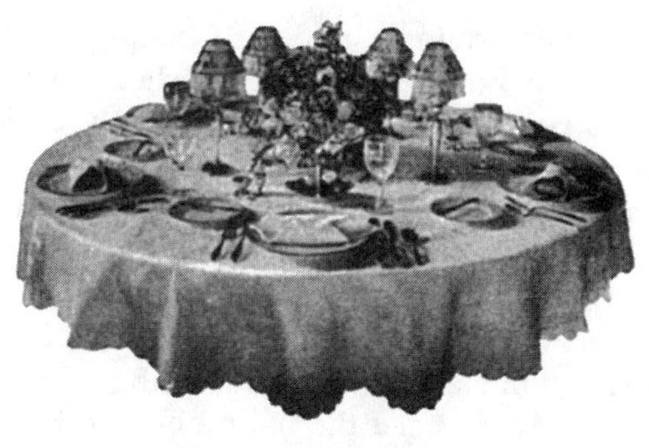

Prologue
Toasted Marshmallows Stuffed with Raisins

In the spring of 1923 a woman wrote to a popular food magazine called *American Cookery* with a question that may have been bothering her for some time:

> Q: Are Vegetables ever served at a buffet luncheon?
>
> A: Yes, indeed . . . provided they appear in a form which will not look messy on the plate. . . . Even the plebian baked bean, in dainty individual ramekins with a garnish of fried apple balls and cress, or toasted marshmallows, stuffed with raisins. . . ."

History almost never records the struggles of anxious middle-class cooks, so it is not possible to know whether this uncertain hostess really did toast a dozen or so marshmallows, pick out their sticky centers, insert a few raisins in each one, and arrange them around ramekins of baked beans; perhaps she settled for the apple balls. But the question and its answer reflect a culinary idealism that held powerful appeal for several generations of American women, beginning in the last quarter of the nineteenth century. This was the era that made American cooking

American, transforming a nation of honest appetites into an obedient market for instant mashed potatoes. The change was remarkably easy to accomplish, although for the women who helped to design and promote it, the pace seemed agonizingly slow and the populace distinctly stubborn. These women lived at a time when science and technology were gaining the aura of divinity: such forces could do no wrong, and their very presence lent dignity to otherwise humble lives and proceedings. Industrialization had already changed the nature of working for one's livelihood; gas and electricity were beginning to change the procedures of daily life; scientists and inventors were bringing forth arresting novelties—the typewriter, the telephone, the light bulb, the calorie—on a regular basis. What chiefly excited these women—an inquisitive circle of ambitious cooks, teachers, writers, and housekeepers—was the link they perceived between science and the world they knew best, the link between science and housework. Traditional methods of housekeeping began to look disturbingly haphazard to them, once they gained an impressionistic understanding of the principles of nutrition and the dangers of germs. Moreover, the very way women approached the day's work seemed irrational and unprofessional compared with the way a well-regulated office or factory could be run. If the home were made a more businesslike place, if husbands were fed and children raised according to scientific principles, if purity and fresh air reached every corner of the house—then, at last, the nation's homes would be adequate to nurture its greatness. Plainly it was their own sister, the unschooled, tradition-bound American housekeeper, who bore responsibility for the failings of the American home, failings that seemed to lead directly to poverty, disease, alcoholism, unemployment, and all the other social miseries apparent at the turn of the century. And by the same reasoning, it was the American housekeeper alone who could guide the nation's homes out of their chaos and into the scientific era. During the last decades of the century, these women engendered a major domestic reform movement, which sprang up in the Northeast and spread rapidly throughout the country. It was known by several names—"scientific housekeeping," "home science," "progressive housekeeping"—but one of the most widely used terms came to be "domestic science." "Looking at the affairs of the household in this new light," wrote a vice-president of one of the national domestic-science organizations, "progressive women have perceived with a growing sense of freedom, how that which has seemed such endless drudgery can, by a clear understanding of underlying principles and the application of scientific methods, be changed into a beautiful harmony of law and order."

This image of primitive domestic labor metamorphosing like a butterfly constituted one of the most appealing messages of the domestic-science movement, and it took on special force in the room where domestic science had its earliest and most important forum: the kitchen. The women who founded and led the domestic-science movement were deeply interested in food, not because they admitted to any particularly intense appetite for it, but because it offered the easiest and most immediate access to the homes of the nation. If they could reform American eating habits, they could reform Americans; and so, with the zeal so often found in educated, middle-class women born with more brains and energy than they were supposed to possess, they set about changing what Americans ate and why they ate it. Some of the cooks in the domestic-science movement inclined toward strict functionalism in the kitchen and others to blatant frivolity—the cuisine they produced under the banner of science could be as dull as a bowl of dry oatmeal or as fanciful as a spring hat—but what united the cooks was their faith in the pragmatic value of each dish. Baked beans surrounded by toasted marshmallows stuffed with raisins would not have been an abomination to any of them, for the combination bespoke major utilitarian sermons. The more self-conscious domestic scientists, the ones who liked to think of themselves as laboratory technicians, would have seen the dish as pedagogical: marshmallows drawing a hesitant populace to the wholly nutritious beans. The juxtaposition of a major protein source such as baked beans with an emblem of pure carbohydrate, moreover, represented to these enthusiasts a rational approach to balancing one's diet, with symbolism so stark the platter might have been a *tableau vivant* of nutritive strategies. Other women, especially the non-professionals who cooked only for their friends and families, would have admired the refining influence of the sweets upon the baked beans. The "plebian" baked bean, old-fashioned and economical, was given new status by being garnished with marshmallows, because sweets were very much a lady's way of assuaging her delicate hunger. To enclose the baked beans in ramekins was to lift them yet another notch in society, for nothing was more repulsive to a refined appetite than food that looked "messy on the plate." With a few raisins the dish became fit to meet the most demanding standards of health and social breeding, and might be expected to exert a pleasing moral influence as well, since a higher-class diet was known to be higher in every sense.

Of necessity, these women were proud of their lifeless palates. The naked act of eating was little more than unavoidable, as far as gently raised women of their era were concerned, and was not to be considered a pleasure except with great discretion. Domestic scientists were inspired by the nutritive properties of food, by its ability to promote physical, social, and, they believed, moral growth. The flavors of food were of slight, somewhat anthropological interest. They did understand very well that many people enjoyed eating; this presented still another challenge. Food was powerful, it could draw forth cravings and greedy desires which had to be met with a firm hand. Their goal as a group was to transubstantiate food, and it didn't matter a great deal whether the preferred method was to reduce a dish to its simplest components or to blanket it with whipped cream and candied violets. Containing and controlling food, draining it of taste and texture, packaging it, tucking the raisins deep inside the marshmallows, decorating it—these were some of the major culinary themes of the domestic-science movement, and they gained credibility far beyond the hopes of the cooks. Americans found a cuisine based on such principles very compatible with their fondness for mechanized and plastic substitutes of all kinds. Frozen peas and onions, packaged in a frozen sauce, never look messy on the plate even after they've been microwaved, and the cooking process that puts the dish on the table may very nearly have taken place, as an old slogan had it, untouched by human hands. Hardly anybody is concerned with the flavor or authenticity of these vegetables—it's the package and the speed that deserve attention. Of course, the domestic scientists, a relatively small group of females, did not re-create the American way of eating all by themselves. On the contrary, they enlisted, and were enlisted by, some of the major institutions of their day: the universities, the public-school system, the government, and the food industry. This combination of influences helped Americans to forget what they once knew about food and to content themselves with convenience, which has long been indistinguishable from progress.

The moment in their history when they turned to institutions for help and legitimation was a crucial one for domestic scientists. Until 1899 they were working in a high-spirited flurry to bring traditional methods of cooking and housekeeping into the twentieth century by opening cooking schools, publishing domestic-science magazines, organizing clubs, and traveling across the country on lecture tours. After that date, which marked the first in a definitive series of domestic-science conferences, they continued all these activities but changed their name and their identity to "home economics." Then they quickly assembled all the appurtenances necessary to a full-fledged profession: syllabi for course work at every level, degree-granting programs of study, a professional organization, a journal, and annual meetings. As home economists, self-anointed professionals, they felt better equipped to tackle a world that still thought of them as a lot of housekeepers with wild ideas. Moreover, they could now join forces with institutions that might help them solidify their position. Home economics easily won a place in industry, education, and government—it won woman's place—and the arrangement satisfied everyone concerned. Home economists were able to convince themselves that these institutions would work to ennoble the American home by modernizing it, and would raise the homemaker to a position of power and dignity by modernizing her as well. Educators greeted home economics as an excellent solution to the insults posed by coeducation, while in government and industry, women who could be trusted to promote the splendors of domesticity—and the necessity to buy new products in order to realize those splendors—were welcomed heartily.

From at least one bleak perspective, the most prominent achievement of the domestic-science movement was the imposition of "home ec" on resentful high-school students everywhere. The ambitious women of the last century who chose cookery as their cause and helped turn the nation toward Wonder Bread hardly qualify as feminist heroines according to the terms of our own time. However passionate, their quest for the germ-free kitchen bears none of the glory we associate with the long struggle for suffrage, birth control, and the rights of citizenship. Yet it would be a mistake to view these women simply as antifeminist throwbacks, or activists gone astray. In truth, their legacy is enormous, albeit by our standards politically unwieldy: it ranges from federal nutrition programs to gelatin salads, and from female chemists to the feminine mystique. Today we are aware of that legacy only insofar as we perceive it in the kind of categories that make sense to us. On the one hand there are scientists, usually male, pursuing important research in nutrition; and on the other hand there are female home economists, teaching schoolgirls how to make baking-powder biscuits. On the one hand there are great chefs, until recently always male; and on the other hand there are women at home, making gravy out of canned soup. On the one hand there are government spokesmen announcing new policies in feeding the poor; and on the other hand there are lunchroom ladies, dishing out exact portions of gray pot roast and boiled carrots in a hot, noisy school cafeteria. But the domestic scientists, who planted the seeds for all these developments, included both extremes at once without regard to caste or tradition or even the rudiments of proportion. They wanted to create a profession for themselves and a creed for women at home, and they wanted to do so by charging ahead into the future. By their reckoning, domestic science was a more radical solution than socialism to the problems of urban poverty, and a more visionary response than feminism to the indignities suffered by women.

The women who chose domestic science had no quarrel with women's rights, but neither did they have any desire to call themselves feminists. They wanted a career and they needed a cause, but they weren't interested in breaking very many rules, reordering society, or challenging men on their own turf. What they really wanted was access to the modern world, the world of science, technology, and rationality, and they believed the best way for women to gain that access was to re-create man's world in woman's sphere. They had no desire to jettison the signs and privileges of middle-class femininity, but liked the notion of a perfectly refined lady with a brisk, manly mind. As they saw it, domestic science would recast women's lives in terms of the future and haul the sentimental, ignorant ways of mother's kitchen into the scientific age. Eventually, and inevitably, the domestic scientists gained second-class citizenship in man's world and died feeling victorious.

The domestic-science movement was a solution for its own time to the same problems ambitious women have always faced. Indeed, the blind faith that characterized the domestic scientists and undermined their idealism is still with us. We live in a time when feminism is considered passé, when rational assessment tells us that all the battles have been won, all the laws are in place, and the only decision women have to make is where to jump aboard. But a hundred years ago people felt exactly the same way. After all, there were laws throughout the country that permitted married women to keep their own earnings; public schools for girls existed in many cities; there were a few female doctors in New York; a female lawyer was arguing cases at the Supreme Court. How much further could society go without embracing total androgyny? The fact that women couldn't vote, that equal pay was an almost unimaginable concept, that birth control was a notorious crime, while rape and wife-beating were best left unmentioned—none of these realities cast much of a shadow on the nation's complacency about free American women, whom patriots liked to contrast with the veiled slaves of the benighted lands of the East. Nowadays, too, successful women can compare themselves with the dimly remembered females of the past and feel smug. They've learned to put feminism behind them, to dress for success, to play the game by men's rules, and to think like men—and they are making the domestic scientists' mistake all over again. There is still a place in every institution for women who think like men, and it's still woman's place.

Their exemplary mistakes are not the only things that make the domestic scientists' story worth telling. What distinguishes them from high-achieving women today and makes them heroines in their own way is their passion. Domestic science was the banner they carried; to change American eating habits was their holy charge; and the recalcitrant nature of the American appetite was their cross. Of course they failed in their crusade, how could they not? They chose domesticity as a way of getting out of the house, and food as a means of transcending the body. But they carved out an identity for women so powerful that we're still trying to clamber out of it, and their influence on American cooking was devastating. They failed, but like only a handful of men and women in any generation, they did their damnedest.

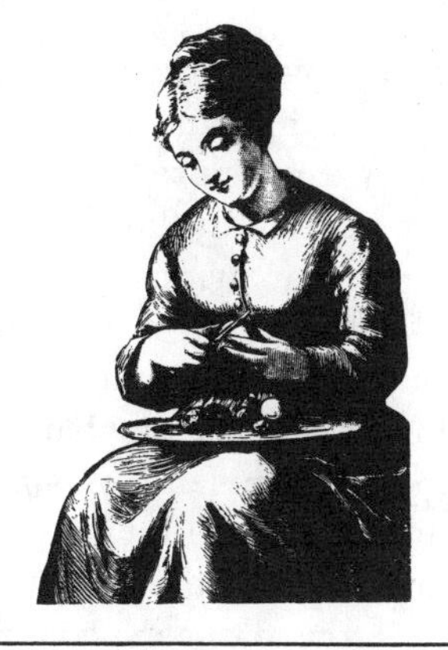

One
Drudgery Divine

Harriet Beecher Stowe once suggested that a special place in heaven be reserved for certain women she called "domestic saints." Her own aunt Esther was a good example—"and her name shall be recorded as Saint Esther"—a spinster who cheerfully gave her life to caring for children, nursing the sick, and silently helping out wherever she saw need. Here was a calling worthy of canonization, wrote Mrs. Stowe: "to be truly noble and heroic in the insipid details of every-day life."

This tribute first appeared in *The Atlantic Monthly* in 1864, a time when home life was considered to be our point of closest contact with heaven. Indeed, the boundary between those two pleasant realms was sometimes indistinct—one best-selling novelist of the day explicitly furnished her heaven with pianos, and provided the angels with gingerbread. Motherhood, of course, best personified the mingling of home and heaven, for a mother was a saint by definition. But while maternity never lost its eminence, during the next few decades an increasing amount of public attention was turned to the actual work involved in home life. Mrs. Stowe's admiration for the righteous doing of "insipid" tasks was one of the earliest signs of what became a national sentiment and finally a mission. "A servant by this clause/Makes drudgery divine/ Who sweeps a floor as for thy laws/Makes that and the action fine," ran a familiar hymn; it was quoted often, in domestic-science classrooms, as a reminder of the divine justification for cooking and cleaning.

The notion of women as emblems of divinity, like the notion of women as emblems of sin, had existed for centuries as a source of comfortable reassurance at least to men. But with the dawn of the industrial age, a volatile economic order gave the old perspective new relevance. Ever since the early 1880s, when industrialization was beginning to transform the country, the question of woman's place in the changing economic and moral scheme of things had been energetically pursued by churchmen, novelists, educators, and popular theoreticians. Women had always been housekeepers and that calling remained their first duty, but housekeeping in the eighteenth century was still an occupation located close to the heart of the economy. Before the effects of technology reached them, women produced nearly everything their families consumed; and these were sizable families that might include visiting relatives and hired help as well as parents and children. The wife, with her daughters and the other women of the house, took charge of spinning, weaving, and sewing, making the family's clothing, linens, and quilts. She gardened and perhaps did some back-yard butchering, made soap and candles, preserved the fruits and vegetables, salted and pickled the meat, churned butter, and baked enormous quantities of bread, pie, and cake. She was responsible for daily housecleaning, weekly laundering and ironing, and major spring and fall cleaning; she was teacher, nurse, doctor, and midwife.

Beginning with the rapid development of textile mills in the early nineteenth century, however, much of the producing and manufacturing work of the household gradually moved outside it. Although technology had little effect on the lives of rural and frontier women until late in the century, by the Civil War period women in the expanding cities and towns were able to buy not only cloth but butter, milk, meat, flour, and myriad household necessities. Schools and hospitals took on the responsibility for teaching children and caring for the seriously sick; and families shrank as the older children and hired help left the household to find work in shops and industries. Even with the resources of a city at hand, however, there was still a great deal of work to do at home. The wife continued to sew and mend, to put three meals a day on the table, and to clean house; while laundry and ironing dominated two or three days of every week. But with the exception of child-rearing, most of the work a woman did consisted of day-to-day maintenance: feeding and cleaning and mending and feeding and cleaning. Her tasks were fewer but they were distinctly monotonous and in a tangible sense unproductive.

The very concept of "work," always a defining feature of man's world, slipped away from woman's, for in the industrial world the value of "work" was measured in cash, while women toiled outside that system. The tasks that women did, moreover, were accomplished very differently from the way industrial work was carried out. The principles of organization and precise scheduling that characterized business and manufacturing were missing from household affairs, which bumped along according to such unpredictable factors as children's tempers and the quality of a batch of yeast. Domestic life was more easily understood as an extension of woman's existence, one of her natural adornments. The best housekeeping, after all, was invisible, offering a smooth surface of cleanliness and harmony that covered up any trace of flurry, mishap, or sweat.

As woman's traditional responsibilities became less and less relevant to a burgeoning industrial economy, the sentimental value of home expanded proportionately. Moralists, theologians, and popular writers produced reams of literature aimed at investing domesticity with the spiritual sweetness of heaven itself. According to these authorities, a woman's most impressive duty was to make her home a heaven in miniature, herself the angel ready at the end of each day to receive and revive the weary worker. This interpretation of her role, while it may not have substituted perfectly for household productivity, did offer a well-defined spiritual challenge to the housekeeper. It was especially pertinent in middle- and upper-class families, where husbands left home each day to dwell in the frankly godless world of commerce and industry—even to profit from it. When they returned home each evening, the most horrifying conditions of factory life and wage-slavery could be gently washed away, all greed absolved, and Christian values brought to the forefront once more, thanks to the domestic angel who spent her day polishing those values into brilliance.

The woman at home came to personify salvation on a daily basis, for the benefit of a society that was still trying to fashion a link between the biblical virtues and worldly success, despite unpleasant evidence to the contrary. Splendid or humble, the domestic hearth became the most grandiose, the most important, the most influential place on earth during this era, because only an image of that immensity could effectively counterbalance the real power of industrialism. Toward the end of the century, this counterbalance would be expressed geographically with the development of suburbs, in which women would pass their days in a world that never met man's world except via public transportation. Around that time, too, the household would come to be recognized as a center of consumption, and the wife as an angel with purchasing power. But the commercialization of home life set into motion at these turning points owed its overwhelming efficiency to the vast amount of moral groundwork performed back in the years before the Civil War. The imagery of Christian sentimentality that blanketed American domestic life in the first decades of the century lent extraordinary new dimensions to the domestic sphere. Popular literature put heaven so close at hand that there were frequent exchanges between the two realms; and in the widely read poetry of that era, dead children would peep down through the clouds to smile at their parents, or God would stop to talk with the woman sweeping the floor of the church. Such easy contact between here and the hereafter, at least at the imaginative level, injected the metaphors of domestic happiness with a vigor they retain even today, especially in the hands of advertisers and politicians.

Women produced copious sentimental literature in these years, not only because they believed the rhetoric, but because this was a professional realm in which they could flourish. Some wrote fiction, some wrote tracts, some wrote hymns, and some edited florid periodicals for ladies—all of which contributed to the establishment of a fairly rigid female culture for nineteenth-century women. By the turn of the century their opulent writing style and dogged moralism were becoming out of date, but the concerns that drove these women to write and sermonize had been taken up by the domestic scientists. As moralists in strictly modern guise, these successors found the link between home and heaven to have been forged by a perfect distribution of proteins, carbohydrates, and fats—they marveled at a divine beneficence that could make the obscure lentil such a resplendent protein source. By maintaining the religious fervor of an earlier generation they were able to put their scientific interests on a pedestal, thus achieving a vantage point that made science more manageable and their pursuit of it more respectable. The charmed partnership between home and heaven that had the early sentimentalists in thrall became an equally charged partnership between home and science. While the domestic scientists never looked back at their literary predecessors with any gratitude—on the contrary, scientific housekeepers learned to despise most evidences of sentimentality in domestic life—it was the moralists, diligently at work through the better part of the nineteenth century, who made it possible for science-minded women to define a sphere for themselves.

The mutual reinforcement between home and heaven

was realized most stirringly in the work of three successful moralists writing at mid-century: Catharine Maria Sedgwick, Elizabeth Stuart Phelps, and Catharine Beecher. In the very different books produced by these women, home life attained such gigantic moral proportions that the progress of civilization itself could be measured according to the rules of domestic propriety. All aspects of home life —the meals, the bed making, the disciplining of naughty children—took on high significance and a heavenly glint, for these were the structures that would keep the nation in order as Americans fulfilled their divine mission: to domesticate the new world. One of the more comprehensive descriptions of how domestic life might pave the way to the everlasting, especially in a newly industrial America, was presented in a straightforward tract by Catharine Maria Sedgwick, who was the well-loved New England author of many moral and historical romances. Miss Sedgwick's didactic purpose led her to enforce a system of rigorous distinctions between right, or uplifting, and wrong, or wholly degrading. The unswerving correctness exemplified in this tract became a kind of moral blueprint for domestic science, which exulted in its freedom from those lackadaisical gray areas lurking between yes and no.

Home, published in 1835 and dedicated to "farmers and mechanics . . . by their friend, the Author," was written by Miss Sedgwick to acquaint the rough, unrefined citizens of the republic with the organizing principles of a rational Christian household. Arranged as a collection of illustrative family scenes, *Home* is dominated by the wisdom of a self-made printer named Mr. Barclay. "Few persons, probably, have thought so much as William Barclay of the economy of domestic happiness," Miss Sedgwick observed. "He had made a chart for his future conduct, by which he hoped to escape at least some of the shoals and quicksands on which others make shipwreck." In the Barclay world there are no awkward moral boundaries dividing commercial from domestic life: the same principles govern each, and Mr. Barclay is the natural steward of both realms. Always vaguely busy at unspecified tasks, Mrs. Barclay provides a silent background of domestic efficiency. It is Mr. Barclay who plans how to govern his household so as to make it an "image of heaven," and Mrs. Barclay who follows a step or two behind, "a loving and, with good reason, a trustful wife. . . ."

The Barclays' real mission in *Home* is to domesticate the whole world, and they begin right after the wedding by furnishing their own little house. Instead of "gewgaws" and "tawdry pictures," they invest in good mattresses and a well-ventilated kitchen, and Mr. Barclay personally selects the books for their new bookcase. This attention to physical and spiritual hygiene benefits everyone who comes in contact with the Barclays. As Miss Sedgwick remarked, "There was a disinfecting principle in the moral atmosphere of their house." Eventually the Barclays have seven children, whom they carefully train in domestic citizenship. The children receive a great deal of their instruction at the family dinner table, for mealtime offers "*three lessons a day,*" Miss Sedgwick emphasized, in a range of virtues including "punctuality, order, neatness, temperance, self-denial, kindness, generosity, and hospitality." At the Barclays' there is no undue concern with the act of eating; rather, the children vie with each other for the pleasure of giving up their favorite food. When only a few strawberries are placed on the table one day—

> "Give mine to Wally, then," said Mary.
>
> "And mine too,—and mine too," echoed and re-echoed from both sides the table.
>
> "And mine too!" repeated little Willie, the urchin next his mother, who had been contentedly eating his potatoe without asking for, or even looking at, the more inviting food on the table.

Little Willie gets no strawberries, not because they are scarce but because Mrs. Barclay believes he is too young to benefit from fruit. Similarly, all the children have been brought up on the plainest food and taught never to ask for anything else. "The monster appetite was thus early tamed," explained Miss Sedgwick. "Its pleasures were felt to be inferior pleasures,—to be enjoyed socially and gratefully, but forbearingly." In addition, these children behave with perfect manners and listen attentively to their elders' conversation. A visitor who drops in during this harmonious meal compares it ruefully with the noisy dinner table he has just left, and concludes that the differences must be chalked up to nature, or perhaps to the failings of his wife. After all, he reminds Mr. Barclay, a man "can't be expected . . . to do much with what you call home education." Mr. Barclay is too polite to correct him. Miss Sedgwick then appends a brief chapter ("The Reverse of the Picture") describing dinnertime at the visitor's own casually run household, where the children fight messily and stuff themselves with rich food, and the parents do no better.

The civilizing function of home is shown on a larger scale when the oldest Barclay son ventures into the wilderness of Ohio to make his living. Charles's new dwelling place is only two rooms but, as he writes to his family, " 'it has quite a home look,' " with its tablecloth embroidered by his sisters, the quilt and curtains also from their hands, the flute, the pile of books. He has been leading prayer services in the settlement, he says, and domesticating the outdoors as well by planting the flowers and fruit trees of his native New England. " 'How soon may we plant a paradise in the wilds, if we will!' " he exclaims. " 'The physical, moral, and intellectual soil is ready; it only wants the spirit of cultivation.' " Shortly afterward Charles catches a fever in Ohio and comes home to die, or actually to make ready his next domicile. Amid the tears and farewells at his deathbed Charles reminds his brothers and sisters that he is only going to a better home, where all of them will meet again as a family in heaven.

Miss Sedgwick rounded out her account of Charles's death with a simple proclamation of faith—"Death has no sting, and the grave no victory, in the home of the Christian"—but even while she wrote, it was becoming noticeable that the religious claims made for domesticity ignored much of the reality of women's lives. What came to be called the "woman movement" surfaced during the years of anti-slavery agitation that preceded the Civil War; and it was the spectacle of the 1840 World's Anti-Slavery Convention—where women delegates were barred from participating—that spurred some of the outraged female abolitionists to identify women's own plight as a cause and to begin to organize around it. In addition, during the last decades of the century the divorce rate was increasing quickly enough to alarm people. Fewer than 10,000 divorces were granted in 1867, but twenty years later there were over 25,000, and at the turn of the century the divorce rate was three times the rate of population growth. Divorce remained a sin and a scandal, but its vivid presence was a reminder of the fragility of domestic bliss. In this period of uncomfortable truth-telling, a young New England woman published the first in a trilogy of novels that presented in the starkest and most powerful terms yet a vision of the household linked to heaven. Elizabeth Stuart Phelps gave new meaning to the concept of a heavenly home by examining it literally: her subject was domestic life after death, and her books on that topic sold in the tens of thousands. Written to comfort, they also managed to criticize—and that edge of bitterness helped to carry the age of domestic sentimentality into the age of domestic science. If Miss Sedgwick wrote the moral blueprint, Elizabeth Stuart Phelps created an emotional blueprint for domestic science: her trilogy on home life in heaven had a passion and a bite that belied its devotional tone and nicely undermined its own air of submission.

Raised in a Calvinist household—her father and grandfather were well-known biblical scholars at Andover Theological Seminary—Miss Phelps received an unusually serious education for a girl in the 1850s, and she also witnessed her mother's painful frustration trying to write books and run a household at the same time. After her mother's early death Miss Phelps grew up with no interest at all in housework ("It was impossible to express . . . her inherent, ineradicable, and sickening recoil from the details of household care," she wrote in one of her several feminist novels), but she retained a great deal of concern with the burdens and rewards of domesticity. The values that distinguished women's work at home—humility, generosity, caring, faith—seemed to her the living fabric of Christianity, and yet they had no very distinguished place in what she called the "cold, smooth theorizing" of the church. In the aftermath of the Civil War, struck by the great suffering of women who had lost husbands and sons, Miss Phelps set out to rescue Christianity from its bloodless male proprietors and turn it over to the real practitioners.

It was an angel, she remarked later, who directed her to write *The Gates Ajar*, the first volume in a unique kind of travel fiction detailing the customs and geography of a wonderful land not very far from New England. The source for this report on heaven is a pleasant woman named Aunt Winifred who arrives to comfort her niece Mary after Mary's treasured brother has been killed in the Civil War. Aunt Winifred's husband is dead, but she is accompanied by her little daughter Faith. After close study of the Bible, and reading numerous commentaries, Aunt Winifred has mapped out an afterlife that horrifies local churchmen and thrills everyone else.

" 'I think I want some mountains,' " she remarks to Mary, " 'and very many trees.' " " 'Mountains and trees!' " gasps her niece. And rivers, brooks, fountains, and flowers will be abundant, Aunt Winifred declares. " 'I hope to have a home of my own,' " she adds. " '. . . In the Father's house are many mansions. Sometimes I fancy that those words have a literal meaning which the simple men who heard them may have understood better than we, and that Christ is truly "preparing" my home for me.' " She goes on to point out that her husband will be there and the two of them will need a place to live. " 'What could be done with the millions who, from the time of Adam, have been gathering there, unless they lived under the conditions of organized society? Organized society involves homes. . . . What other arrangement could be as pleasant or could be pleasant at all?' "

The personification of Aunt Winifred's faith is, of course, Faith, not at all the dogged, Job-like hero of the usual tracts and sermons, but a rough-and-tumble three-year-old who plays outdoors in the mud all day and constantly gets into mischief. She and Aunt Winifred discuss heaven frequently, and Faith in turn entertains her playmates with the news. " 'P'r'aps I'll have some strawberries, too, and some ginger-snaps,—I'm not going to have any old bread and butter there,—O, and some little gold apples, and a lot of playthings; nicer playthings—why, nicer than they have in the shops in Boston, Molly Bland! God's keeping 'em up there a purpose.' " In like manner, Aunt Winifred is able to assure a talented neighborhood girl that in heaven she will have the piano that she longed for on earth, and she brightens a stolid country boy by advising him that he might be able to operate machinery in heaven. " 'I don't see how *I'm* going to wear white frocks and stand up in a choir,—never could sing more'n a frog with a cold in his head,' " muses the boy. " 'Perhaps I could help 'em build a church, hist some of their pearl gates, or something like!' "

This domestic theology deeply shocks the clergymen in town, whose pointed names are Dr. Bland and Deacon Quirk. Both are fond of depicting heaven in its traditional terms—angelic choirs playing harps and crying "Worthy the Lamb!" The death of his wife in a kitchen fire, however, thrusts Dr. Bland onto another level of feeling. As the agonized woman is on her deathbed, unable to stop thinking of the four little children she is leaving motherless, Aunt Winifred confides to her that she isn't really leaving them motherless at all, that God will make it possible for her to take care of them even from above. Finally at ease, the woman allows herself to die peacefully. Dr. Bland has a long talk with Aunt Winifred, and some time later Mary notes in her journal that he seems very changed. "A certain indefinable *humanness* softens his eyes and tones, and seems to be creeping into everything he says."

Not surprisingly, Aunt Winifred herself dies at the end of the book, painfully but gladly expiring from breast cancer while Faith romps about the bedside. Aunt Winifred's last act is to look toward the window and greet her husband. And in the next two volumes, while the characters change, Miss Phelps makes it clear that Aunt Winifred was right in her assumptions, and the Quirks and Blands quite wrong. In *Beyond the Gates* and *The Gates Between* Miss Phelps takes up the day-to-day life of two newcomers in heaven—a woman in the second volume and a man in the third—whose experiences differ significantly. The woman is delighted with heaven: she loves the little cottage she is given, she goes to a concert featuring a new oratorio by Beethoven (his hearing has been restored), and meets a great many artists, poets, and scientists. She also meets God—and he is very much a woman's God. No thunderbolts, no wrath, no mighty judge, this God is just an unusually nice man who falls into conversation with her one day, lets her do most of the talking, and actually listens. Afterward she feels as though she has found a friend, her best friend ever. Perhaps the strongest indication that heaven is a woman's world comes at the moment when the heroine—who was unmarried on earth—begins to feel as lonely in heaven as she used to feel in life. "The old ache has survived the grave," she thinks. Just then she comes across the man she had loved years ago, who married another woman and found out his mistake too late. Now, at last, he can marry the heroine—for in this world view a mistake of that importance mercifully ends with death and can be rectified afterward for eternity. God himself blesses the new union, lest it strike any reader as uncomfortably close to bigamy.

Everything that pleases a woman in heaven is appalling to the man who arrives there in the last book, *The Gates Between*. He is a busy doctor who has died right after hurling some mean, thoughtless words at his devoted wife, and when he gets to heaven he wanders around feeling frustrated and confused. "It is all unfamiliar to me," he complains. "I am afraid I have not been educated for it. It is the most unhomelike place I ever saw." Eventually he does learn to make a heavenly home, but not until he has been educated in the values of domesticity. The sudden death and arrival in heaven of his son forces the doctor to set up a household and to care for the little boy. When he goes out to look for work, however, he finds he is not qualified to be a physician in heaven. "Here in this world of spirits I was an unscientific, uninstructed fellow," he admits; and takes a lowly job in maintenance, cleaning up at the heavenly hospital. Finally, in response to the innocent promptings of his little son, he begins to teach himself the more important sciences of love and faith. Then his ambition increases: he decides to request a new job as a spiritual healer in earthly homes. "I wished to . . . set the whole force of a man's experience and a spirit's power to make an irritable scene in loving homes held as degrading as a blow. . . ." With this awareness his education is complete, and he is rewarded by the arrival of his wife and the establishment of a familiar, but greatly improved, domestic circle in heaven.

With *Beyond the Gates* and *The Gates Between* Miss Phelps made it clear that the distance between earthly and heavenly domestic life was greater than popular rhetoric might admit. A home free of anger, loneliness, and pain was not going to spring up easily around every family, even a loving family. Truly blessed domesticity could only be achieved through devotion and self-sacrifice, as the doctor learns; and the way he learns is by taking up the humble occupations of women.

Twenty years after creating the ideal world of *Home* Catharine Maria Sedgwick also came around to depicting a few of the pressures on domestic happiness. In *Married or Single?* a couple somewhat less perfect than the Barclays is carefully running a Christian household with the husband firmly positioned at the head of the family. One morning he speaks harshly to his wife at the breakfast table, and later in the day he apologizes. With her usual benevolence his wife tells him that when he is in a bad temper she simply thinks of him as another baby in the house, who must be diverted and soothed. Furthermore, she adds, "'. . . these little trials are mere exhalations from the ground, that melt away in the sunshine of our love; . . . you are my teacher, my master, my daily bread.'" This wifely attitude leads Miss Sedgwick to comment approvingly: "With more of such Christian unions there would be fewer divorces for 'incompatibility,' and a long lull to the stormy question of 'women's rights.'"

Miss Sedgwick never married, which undoubtedly made it easier for her to praise domesticity so comfortably as its own reward. Miss Phelps, however, married late and unhappily, and her painful understanding of wifely self-sacrifice was made clear in the openly feminist novels she began to produce after *The Gates Ajar*. Both these experts in divine domesticity, then, recognized the gap between the rhetoric and the reality of domestic life. It was their different perspectives on how best to close that gap that symbolized the threats and opportunities faced by women raised on pure sentimentality. Miss Phelps tended to blame men for most domestic disruption, and would have liked them to take on some of the female qualities of humility, generosity, and moral wisdom. At the level of allegory Miss Sedgwick felt the same way—Mr. Barclay is virtually female in his goodness—but in what passed for realistic fiction she accepted as unchangeable the fact that sometimes a husband was just another baby in the house. Miss Phelps's acknowledgment of the bitter problems that maleness could create, both theologically and domestically, helped women of her time to see more clearly through the fog of nineteenth-century religiosity, but relatively few of them saw straight through to feminism. Outright challenge to the male was never a widespread solution to the domestic difficulties of the postwar era; instead, women developed ways to maneuver within accepted boundaries. Most often, married women with some free time joined clubs for self-betterment or threw themselves into dozens of projects and causes they could construe as beneficial to someone else. Even in this activist frame of mind, however, many clung to the attitude represented by Miss Sedgwick: that women had a special responsibility to ensure the success of domestic life. This mix of traditional responsibilities with a new reforming spirit helped give rise to domestic science, the movement that enabled women to focus critical attention not on their husbands but on their housework.

For the domestic scientists, criticizing domestic life meant glossing over its contradictions and confusions, imposing order upon chaos, and polishing the surface—a systematic program of sanitation that apparently operated on their own public personalities as well as their households. Domestic scientists loved to create models of the ideal housekeeper, their modern woman—someone serene, unhurried, and with a mind fixed on eternal truths, who would move through a day of chores and challenges like an invisible force for good, applying the laws of chemistry and biology to every mark of disarray. Not until fairly late in the movement, as it was becoming home economics and trying to establish its validity as a profession, did domestic scientists finally acknowledge their history and discover that Catharine Beecher had been there ahead of them. In Miss Beecher's 1841 best-seller, *A Treatise on Domestic Economy*, the image of the ideal American housekeeper leading her family and hence the nation into a glorious Christian future was delineated in every particular, from diagrams of the skeletal system to suggestions for charitable beekeeping. Unlike Miss Sedgwick and Miss Phelps, Catharine Beecher took a lively interest in the details of housekeeping: for her, domesticity really did mean scrubbing and boiling and ironing and darning, not to mention architecture, plumbing, and agriculture. Yet her perspective was anything but narrow: she preferred to discuss female domesticity in what she considered its most meaningful context—the progress of America—and worked to put housekeeping on an intellectual level that would match its moral loftiness. *A Treatise on Domestic Economy* was an early blueprint for the domestic scientist herself, the woman educated for acquiescence who would re-create heaven on earth by attending to the surface of things, perpetually inspired by her accommodation to a higher authority.

Born in 1800, Catharine Beecher grew up a brainy, energetic woman in a family devoted to men. The Beecher patriarch was Lyman Beecher, the famous evangelical preacher, and he concentrated the family resources on sending his sons to college and seminary so that they, too, might become ministers. His daughters were raised to become wives—preferably the wives of ministers—and to care for them as assiduously as Lyman Beecher's three wives each cared for him. As the oldest of thirteen children Catharine Beecher learned early on to help keep house and raise children. Following some decorous schooling and a brief, unchallenging teaching job, she dutifully fell in love with a young science professor at Yale. Her fiancé died in a shipwreck before they could marry, however, and she appears never to have seriously contemplated another engagement. After his death she spent some time going over his scientific papers, and took his place briefly as tutor to his younger sisters—an experience that set her life in an altogether new direction. Teaching herself algebra, geometry, chemistry, and other branches of science, in order to understand his work and to teach his sisters, Catharine Beecher discovered that she had an excellent mind and loved using it. In 1823 she opened her first school, the Hartford Female Seminary, and she spent the rest of her life gathering converts to her chosen cause: women's education.

Teaching and running a school were suitable enough pursuits for a young spinster, but Catharine Beecher had a great deal more ambition than any single job could satisfy. After seven years at Hartford she left her thriving school and set out on a career that would keep her traveling among the major cities, in constant touch with educational leaders, writers, thinkers, and philanthropists. The vision she was promoting took different forms at different times in her career, but in essence she saw the

American woman as Teacher: the teacher in the family circle, the teacher in school, and the moral teacher for the whole burgeoning republic as it led civilization toward an exalted future. All these dreams for American women started in the same place: the founding of a great training institution for women that would be financially endowed, just as men's were. Catharine Beecher worked vigorously to raise funds and win the support of wealthy people for her projects, but none of the schools she planned took shape as she wished; and again and again she would end her involvement by abandoning them and moving on to her next idea. A prolific writer of books, pamphlets, and articles, she supported herself through the sale of her domestic manuals, and it was these immensely successful volumes that established her credibility during her lifetime and assured her reputation afterward.

A Treatise on Domestic Economy appeared in 1841, seven years before the first women's rights convention was held at Seneca Falls, New York; but Catharine Beecher's exhaustive analysis of woman's role had little in common with the Female Declaration of Independence that was to emerge from Seneca Falls. It was not that she was unaware of the legal, educational, and social deprivations that American women endured—like many of the women at Seneca Falls, she had watched her brothers go off to college while she stayed home to do the laundry and mending they sent back—but she painstakingly spelled out a way to accommodate those deprivations, rather than confront them. Along with her detailed instructions for running a household, she offered a new identity for the American woman in which conflict had no part and sex inequalities were transformed into a manifestation of God's blessing on his favored republic. The image of woman she promulgated in her introductory chapter ("Peculiar Responsibilities of American Women") was not very much like her own argumentative and strong-minded self; on the contrary, it was an image that closed off argument, smoothed over any abrasive questions, and rounded any sharp edges of a woman's personality.

Anticipating the era of huge, encyclopedic manuals, *A Treatise on Domestic Economy* was surely among the most comprehensive even by later standards. One of the few authors to write out directions for tying the bedsheets together and lowering oneself out the window when the house is on fire, Catharine Beecher had a commitment to thoroughness and a distinct bent for detail. Although her book came out less than a decade after Lydia Maria Child's *The American Frugal Housewife*, hitherto the most popular domestic manual written for Americans, Catharine Beecher's was a different and much more sophisticated undertaking. Mrs. Child collected recipes and household hints that would have been useful in any well-run home: how to make limewater in which to preserve eggs for up to three years, how to clear the house of red ants, how to prepare a home vapor-bath, how to make cheap custards. In addition, Mrs. Child featured plainspoken essays on the importance of thrift and good work habits. Her advice was not scholarly—indeed, some of it bordered on the superstitious—but it was certainly practical. She urged families of moderate income to avoid traveling, for example, especially pleasure trips to such fashionable spots as Niagara and Quebec, for not only was it an expensive amusement of no lasting value but the acquaintances one visited en route might well turn up themselves the next summer, fully expecting to be housed and entertained. *The American Frugal Housewife* remained a reassuring favorite, but it represented a distinctly old-fashioned approach to home life, and *A Treatise on Domestic Economy* overlapped very little with it.

Catharine Beecher was interested in promoting not only the right way but the right reason, and her elaborate justification for the "peculiar responsibilities" of her sex soared to nationalism and beyond. The legal subordination of American women, she argued carefully, was actually an important feature of democracy, for it ensured that the principle of equality would reign over the nation. In a country where all were equal, certain controls had to be established to prevent selfish interests from interrupting the administration of the general good. God, the "Supreme Lawgiver," had created a model for such controls in the relationship of parent to child; and in like manner, the employer must be held superior to the employed, the teacher to the pupil, and the husband to the wife. Moreover, while woman's equal benefit from all civic, social, and political matters was not in dispute, in America "it is decided that" these privileges were best secured for her by being entrusted to men. Therefore she need not vote, or participate in government. The smooth functioning of American society was assured under this system. Its fairness could be contrasted with the English way, in which poverty and ignorance were the lot of many, "that a few may live in palaces and riot in every indulgence." America had been chosen, in fact, to be a beacon to such nations—"already the light is streaming into the dark prison-house of despotic lands"—and to spread Christianity and democracy throughout the world. In this great work, the American woman was blessed with a special task. In her capacity as mother, sister, and wife she would mold men's characters so as to affect the whole moral and intellectual configuration of society. "Let the women of a country be made virtuous and intelligent, and the men will certainly be the same," Catharine Beecher charged. And here she included the message that always accompanied her most fervent preaching: "The proper education of a man decides the welfare of an individual; but educate a woman, and the interests of a whole family are secured."

Catharine Beecher always emphasized that domestic labor should be studied by all young girls, rich and poor, so that the impression might soon spread that these pursuits were "refined and lady-like" rather than mere "drudgery" and "dirty work" best left to servants. "It is because such work has generally been done by vulgar people, and in a vulgar way, that we have such associations," she noted, "and when ladies manage these things, as ladies should, then such associations will be removed." The concept of refined housekeeping, which would become such a prominent motif in domestic science, received its first substantial analysis here. Of course Catharine Beecher was not implying that ladies should simply fire the "vulgar people" they employed, but rather that every lady should understand every household process so that she might properly teach her servants. In addition, because of the unpredictable economic conditions in American life, she argued that every woman should be able to assume all household chores with full confidence the moment her husband lost his fortune, or her servant ran off to work in a mill. Under any circumstances, moreover, the lady of the house would be responsible for maintaining the family's health, raising the children, and keeping the household on an efficient daily schedule. Nor was it beyond the scope of her management to oversee gardens, orchards, and yards, architecture and construction of the home, plumbing and ventilation, and the care of horses, sows, dogs, cats, and poultry. "It may, at first glance, appear that this kind of knowledge is not needed by a woman," Catharine Beecher conceded as she began her chapter on animals and barns. "But how often it is the case, that the death or absence of a husband, or a father, throws all the care of a whole establishment on a woman." An emphasis on self-sufficiency always distinguished her definition of the ladylike.

Self-sufficiency, self-control, and a perfectly bland façade were the most prominent features of the well-trained homemaker as Catharine Beecher saw her, and although all but self-sufficiency were personally foreign to her, she included chapters on "Domestic Manners," "Good Temper in a Housekeeper," and "Habits of System and Order," all designed to free the homemaker and the household from hurry, waste, and chaos. Acknowledging the distractions and annoyances that constantly interfered with daily housekeeping, Catharine Beecher explained that the surest way to maintain harmony and calm was to keep one's mind fixed upon the greatness of the work itself. Every woman should be trained from childhood to believe that hers were "the most important, the most difficult, and the most sacred and interesting duties that can possibly employ the highest intellect." Holding fast to this outlook she could apportion her time and take up each task systematically, knowing that interruptions were inevitable but aware, too, that even a burnt pudding or a badly swept room was "appointed by Perfect Wisdom" and controlled by a Heavenly Parent.

As a kind of Heavenly Parent herself, Catharine Beecher placed special emphasis on the elements of house construction in her manuals, thus ensuring that what she called "habits of system and order" might be literally built into every home. For her, a woman's mastery of house construction was tantamount to mastering a way to live. The houses she designed and recommended were models not only of economy and efficiency but of moral certainty, as if she were trying to realize a domestic citizenship that had no counterpart in the outside world. For "persons of moderate circumstances," especially young wives and mothers in their first years of homemaking, she recommended an ingenious cottage organized around two main rooms and a kitchen, but capable, by means of various disguised beds, of sleeping as many as eight people with adequate ventilation for all. This house had the orderly proportions of a tidy classical temple and should, she emphasized, be painted white. In another house, larger than the first but where "most of the domestic labor is to be performed by the ladies of the family," the dining room is dispensed with and a single large room for cooking and eating takes its place. Again, a certain amount of discreet hiding was called for. In this early version of the eat-in kitchen, the sink and oven were located in a small adjoining room, so that laundry, baking, and dishwashing—"the most soiling employments"—need not occur where the family ate, or within anyone's sight.

While every home she designed was planned with economy in mind, particularly economy of labor, she did increase the scale significantly for families in grander circumstances, and the more spacious these homes became, the more their exteriors resembled houses of worship. Her most resplendent house suggested a small cathedral. The culmination of this theme appeared in one of her last volumes, *The American Woman's Home*, in which she showed a house neatly capped with its own steeple and cross. This dwelling was built to double as a neighborhood school during the week and a church on Sunday, and it gave tangible form to Catharine Beecher's long-held belief that the American woman was the nation's best educator and religious guide. While later domestic scientists would treat the same concept metaphorically, Catharine Beecher provided diagrams and work plans. This would be the definitive home for what she called the "Christian family" in the "Christian neighborhood"; and here, in the last decade of her life, she took the remarkable step of portraying the "highest kind of 'Christian family' " as a family of women. Two or three women might live together, she proposed, and take in a few of the sick and destitute, or raise orphans, or train deprived young boys and girls in healthy, outdoor employments such as horticulture and beekeeping. This picture, saturated though it was in her most evangelical prose, offered a comfortable version of female leadership and self-sufficiency that plainly held tremendous appeal for Catharine Beecher. She never disavowed her belief in the subordinate, protected status of women, and she always took pleasure in her own family as well as constant visits with other families; yet she had committed herself early to spinsterhood. There is no evidence that she regretted that choice, but it left her a perpetual guest, on the fringe of any domestic circle. Many single women attached themselves as helpful aunts to one or another family household, but Catharine Beecher was too independent for that sort of existence. In her image of the highest kind of Christian family she conjured up a deeply satisfying life in which a respectable woman could enjoy domesticity and still control her own days and destiny.

That same elusive balance between domesticity and independence lured many women to the domestic-science movement, which appealingly enough called for a change of imagery—the technician was to replace the angel—but not a change of belief. These women would keep to women's sphere but try to redefine it, try to cleanse domestic life of its disappointments. During the years that Miss Sedgwick, Miss Phelps, and Miss Beecher were writing on divine domesticity, a growing array of experts on earthly domesticity began publishing abundant directions for the task.

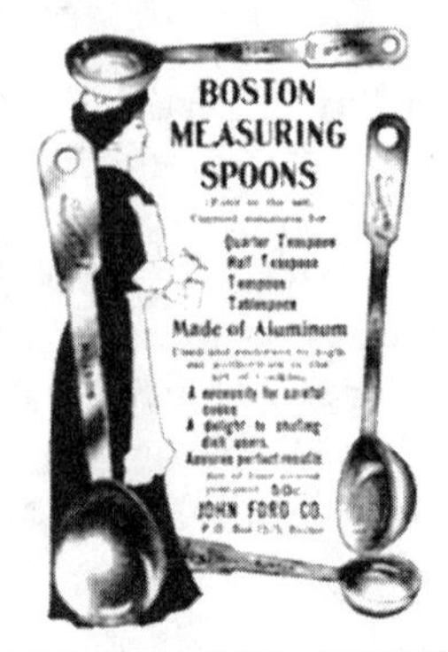

Two

And the Kitchen Becomes the Workshop of the Skies

" 'I have been keeping house a number of years but somehow my home is never as tidy as other people's,' " complained a reader of the *Ladies' Home Journal* in a letter to that magazine's housekeeping department. Dozens of similar letters received by the magazine were summarized by a housekeeping editor over the course of a few months:

"Lives on a farm and has the 'best husband in the world' but the work is never done and the meals can never be served daintily as she had planned before she was married because they must always 'hurry, hurry.' "

"Has been married three years but can't grasp the idea of managing her home."

"Is so young and inexperienced that the servant girls walk all over her."

" 'Please map out a housecleaning campaign.' "

"How to serve dessert when there is no maid—'it is so tiresome and confusing to clear away everything and then bring in the dessert.' "

"Woman does all the work including laundry for a family of ten—is obliged to carry all the water that is used in the house—are there any efficiency methods that would help?"

" 'My kitchen work always seems like drudgery.' "

Cookbooks, etiquette guides, housekeeping texts, and mother's manuals were pouring onto the market at the turn of the century, and women's magazines were filled with much the same information, all of it supporting the image of home as a refuge for men but a lifelong challenge for women. There were rules available to guide a woman through every moment of her day, and looming behind every rule in this careful delineation of work methods was the persistent threat of failure. Hurry, confusion, disorganization—a domestic chaos always hovered just out of sight, ready to descend as soon as a mattress was left unturned or the oatmeal was insufficiently cooked. It was woman's job to stave off that chaos, to rescue her family every day in a thousand little ways from the dirt and disorder that signaled disaster. "Is it not pitiful, this army of incompetent wives," exclaimed a New York member of a domestic-science association, "whose lack of all knowledge of domestic science is directly and indirectly the means of filling our prisons, asylums, reformatories and saloons!" The air itself carried invisible poisons, and the "disinfecting principle" Miss Sedgwick had praised in the moral atmosphere of the Barclay household now had to be understood literally. "Suppose my cellar is a dark, ill ventilated, damp hole, what follows?" asked a cleaning expert rhetorically in the pages of *Good Housekeeping*. "Silently, by day and by night, the moisture creeps up the walls, pervades the whole atmosphere of the house, enters every closet and sleeping compartment, and soon the physician is called; the family is being troubled with sore throats, rheumatism appears . . . then diphtheria and fevers follow, and at last death comes. . . ."

This image of barely averted chaos did more than lend a moral urgency to the drama of housekeeping: it called for women to seize control of their surroundings, perhaps for the first time in their lives. Raised to feel dependent—

even, if they could afford it, completely helpless—most women had little opportunity to influence their own destinies. After the Industrial Revolution, moreover, women could not even be assured of marrying into a predictable future. Any family might be subjected to sudden swings between comfort and poverty, and women who had been taught to keep their distance from financial matters were unprepared for changes of income in either direction. Increasingly, too, women were leaving their familiar worlds behind when they married and traveling hundreds of miles to set up housekeeping in new cities, far from the mothers, aunts, and friends who had always been the best sources of domestic advice and support. The isolation and frustration that accompanied these marriages were portrayed constantly in stories that ran in the housekeeping magazines. " 'Nearly every young housekeeper has a spell of left-handed housekeeping, and some never get over it,' " explains an aunt who comes to visit for a week in one of these stories. Her newly married niece has just pulled a loaf of bread from the oven without a pot holder, burnt her fingers, sent a china teapot crashing to the floor, and burst into tears. The aunt has been watching such catastrophes all week, and invites her niece to sit down for some guidance. " 'You were in too much of a hurry and took chances,' " she begins. " 'You should have found your holder or taken something equally good for handling hot tins. Then, the teapot ought to have been washed and put away when you washed the dishes. . . .' " Gratefully the young bride listens, and concludes by resolving, " 'I'm going to be a good housekeeper and homekeeper first of all, and then, when Charlie's salary is raised and we can afford to keep a girl, I shall know how things ought to be done.' "

Such an approach to housework, by way of rules and schedules, was meant to impose a sense of manageability over the day's work and make the actual toil all but invisible. The "ideal housekeeper," as the author of *Progressive Housekeeping* put it, was "the one who, without seeming to give much heed to the wheels of her household machinery, has it in such perfect running order that it seems to go of itself." By way of contrast, the author went on to describe what she called a more familiar type, the old-fashioned "strenuous housekeeper." Anxiety haunts the days and nights of this unfortunate; she has no real control over her work, for "if her eye and hand are withdrawn chaos reigns." The difference between these two housekeepers, all authorities agreed, was a matter of education. Under the scrutiny of persistent study and discussion, domesticity expanded into an objective body of knowledge that had to be actively pursued; it was no longer to be treated as a God-given expertise insensibly commanded by all women. The most popular way to refer to this approach was to call it "scientific." Indeed, one of the most impressive ways to describe anything in the latter half of the nineteenth century was to call it scientific, and terms like "scientific motherhood," "scientific charity," and "scientific cookery" were in constant use whenever women analyzed their modern responsibilities. By scientific they meant rational, objective, and methodical—traits that gave the term a definite air of maleness. "A man must be thoroughly acquainted with the details of his business to make his business a success," pointed out a Chautauqua cooking teacher. "It is equally true in regard to the occupations in which women engage. . . . No woman is fitted to be a wife or mother, or to preside over a home, who has not a practical knowledge of household science." Scientific housekeeping, its proponents liked to suggest, demanded the rigorous intellect and objectivity of a man's mind. This was never taken to mean that men ought to do housework, of course; the point was that women had to be trained to think like men.

The woman who worked hardest to appropriate male thinking into the feminine domain was Ellen Richards, one of the founders of domestic science both as a reform movement and as a world view, and perhaps its best-loved leader. Ellen Richards was the first woman to cross into man's scientific world and return with good news for housekeepers. A Vassar graduate, she applied to the Massachusetts Institute of Technology in 1870 and was admitted as a "special student"—special because the institute had never before admitted a woman and was deeply hesitant about this one. Aware that she was an experiment, she volunteered to sweep the laboratory floor and sew on buttons for her professors all during her student years. This approach, she wrote to her parents, made her a good deal more acceptable than if she had been a "Radical." The same conscientious effort to juggle her allegiances was maintained throughout her long career; indeed, the uneasy jostling between her own predilections and her vision of perfect womanhood made Ellen Richards a latter-day Catharine Beecher. While she was still a student she agreed to teach a woman's chemistry course, which the Woman's Education Association had set up in a local high school for lack of any other opportunities in Boston for women to gain entrance to a chemistry laboratory. Following her graduation, Mrs. Richards came up with an ingenious and polite way to raise the academic level of this course and introduce more women into the institute. If the WEA would provide funds to set up and equip a full-fledged chemistry laboratory for women, MIT would house it in one of its temporarily unused buildings. The Woman's Laboratory opened in 1876, with Mrs. Richards and an institute professor in charge—both of them volunteering their services, since there were no funds for salaries—and they trained dozens of women every year until 1884, when MIT agreed to incorporate women as regular students.

Mrs. Richards devoted a great deal of professional and personal time to the Woman's Laboratory, and donated thousands of dollars to its maintenance. For the most part her students were women already in teaching positions who had had no access to the study of chemistry while they were in school. But she also intended the laboratory to establish " 'new and wider fields for women's work in the professional branches of applied chemistry. . . .' " Nonetheless, women's most ground-breaking work in applied chemistry, as Mrs. Richards saw it, was a specialty she had developed herself called Household Chemistry. In this course women made chemical analyses of different kinds of baking soda, vinegar, and spices, not only to know their composition, but to learn how to identify adulterated products. In addition they studied the chemical processes involved in cooking and digesting food, raising bread, and cleaning different fabrics and surfaces. Mrs. Richards did more than simply channel her students in this direction: she ran her own home as if it were an extension of the Woman's Laboratory, and conducted regular tests on the products and technologies introduced into her housekeeping. She called her house in the outlying neighborhood of Jamaica Plain the "center for right living," and hoped it would exemplify the way in which the highest scientific standards could enhance daily life if they were applied to eating, sleeping, breathing, house construction, housecleaning, and home decoration.

Outside the classroom and the household, Mrs. Richards carried out significant research in the chemistry of sanitation, water analysis, and fire prevention, both at MIT and as a consultant to private industry. She took a generous interest in her students' work as well, and assisted many young women into professional careers of their own. But the heroine of her best-known writing and thinking was always the woman at home, and it was to promote and magnify the role of the housekeeper that Mrs. Richards became one of the chief organizers and theoreticians of the domestic-science movement. "Woman was originally the inventor, the manufacturer, the provider," she explained in an article aimed at bright, but listless, housewives. "She has allowed one office after another gradually to slip from her hand, until she retains, with loose grasp, only the so-called housekeeping. . . . Having thus given up one by one the occupations which required knowledge of materials and processes, and skill in using them . . . she rightly feels that what is left is mere deadening drudgery. . . ."

The solution she proposed to this particular audience was a lengthy reading course for home study in domestic science, and she listed handbooks on bacteria and sanitation, plumbing and house construction, cleaning and cooking methods, nutrition, food adulteration, and diet for the sick. These suggestions, she emphasized, were meant to "help the housewife to regain control over her kingdom." The theme of woman's kingdom slowly slipping away from her, of men appropriating woman's work and removing it to the industrial world outside the home, was a recurring one in Mrs. Richards's lectures and articles. "Was she beguiled by flattery to sell her birthright?" she wondered aloud before an audience of Ohio college women. "Whatever the reason, we find ourselves now in a desperate case. . . . The fact is that the industrial world is ruled by science and that all the things with which we surround ourselves are now manufactured upon scientific principles, and, alas! women are ignorant of those principles." Mrs. Richards did believe that science, technology, and industry were doing a much better job of assuring the family's health and safety than most mothers could, but she was unwilling to conclude that nothing at all remained of women's old-fashioned domestic role. Home was still, above all, an oasis, a retreat from the bustle of the world; and to maintain its soothing atmosphere of peace was still the responsibility of the mistress of the household. Surrendering this ideal of family life, Mrs. Richards asserted, would be a "long step toward socialistic communism."

Ellen Richards's career, which began in the 1870s and was still going strong when she stepped down from the presidency of the American Home Economics Association in 1910, shortly before her death, marked the transition between pure domesticity, an abiding virtue, and domestic science, the new profession. Most of the domestic scientists who set the movement on its course during these decades either were trained by Ellen Richards or worked alongside her, or at the very least owned a copy of her first book, *The Chemistry of Cooking and Cleaning*, which remained in steady demand for close to thirty years. Inspired by Mrs. Richards's zeal and energy these women launched themselves in every direction open to them, teaching and writing and lecturing first in New England and soon across the country. They organized the Cooking Teachers' League, the

National Household Economic Association, and numerous local housekeepers' clubs; they started magazines devoted to housekeeping and cooking; and they built up cooking schools and degree programs in domestic science in all the major cities. "We need to exalt the profession of home making," an editorial in *New England Kitchen Magazine* said bluntly, "to see that it is as dignified and requires as much intelligence as other professions." When an unnamed "literary woman" charged in a popular weekly magazine that the science of housekeeping could be mastered by any woman of normal intelligence in six weeks, the editors of *American Kitchen Magazine* sprang to the challenge. Fifty letters were sent to "representative women," asking whether the statement was true, and a selection of their replies was published. "If the piano or violin can be learned in six weeks, so can housekeeping," was Ellen Richards's acid comment. Cooking teacher Maria Parloa thought that a year might be sufficient; other women reported that seventeen years, or twenty, or fifty, had not been long enough for them to feel they had thoroughly mastered their work. "If a woman is well educated, has a knowledge of chemistry and can adapt it to the requirements of cooking, cleaning, laundry work, hygiene and sanitation of the home, if she knows how to care for clothing and house linen, all about germs and dust, plumbing and sewage, how to care for floors and furniture; if she has a thorough knowledge of the various foods, the economic, scientific and nutritive value of the same, with infinite patience I think she could master the minor details of the science of housekeeping in about six weeks," summed up a woman doctor from Michigan.

The new domestic heaven they were promoting was a household that ran as quietly and productively as a machine, under the guidance of a benevolent technician. There was only one major obstacle, as far as most leaders of the movement could see, and that was women themselves. Most American wives seemed to be stuck in the past, unable to envision housework as anything but a wearisome daily round. They were likely to impede the progress of the nation simply because they refused to imagine themselves operating the home laboratory of the future. A writer in *New England Kitchen Magazine* pleaded for women to open their minds to the new labor-saving inventions, which, she noted, were valued only by those few women with the "industrial spirit." The average housewife, she stressed, was afraid and mistrustful of the new clothes washers, dishwashers, and gas and electric stoves. "The daily treadmill gone through in a mechanical fashion with little mental effort is stultifying; introduce the factor of machinery and an awakening is inevitable," she urged. "One feels a peg higher in the scale of intelligence for using even a dishwashing machine. . . ." The term most frequently employed when domestic scientists criticized old-fashioned, uneducated housekeeping was "drudgery," which not only described the endless round of housework itself but suggested a lack of enlightenment on the part of the housekeeper. "The woman who boils potatoes year after year, with no thought of the how or why, is a drudge," Ellen Richards explained to the Association of Collegiate Alumnae, "but the cook who can compute the calories of heat which a potato of given weight will yield, is no drudge."

For many domestic scientists, the easiest way to combat a persistently bleak popular image of housework was to call upon its old redemptive factor, which still lent the glow of the select to any housekeeper and gave stature to woman's work. "From lowly tasks abundant honors rise, and the kitchen becomes the workshop of the skies," observed a Midwestern clubwoman, concluding an essay on "The Ethics of the Kitchen." Housework was a science, but a particularly beneficent science; a career, but an especially feminine career; a branch of technology, but an exalted one marked out for women. The degrading identification of housework with servants' work was hard to erase, but domestic scientists did their best to underscore the dignity and respectability of home tasks no matter where in the social order they might be performed. Anna Barrows, who edited *New England Kitchen Magazine* with Mary J. Lincoln, suggested in the course of a lecture on "The Apple in Cookery" that women who had to earn their livings might consider making crystallized apples to sell. With suitable training, she remarked, any woman could make a living preparing these "dainty confections" in her own home. "Would not such an occupation be more desirable than 'sale' work?" asked Miss Barrows. Making and selling crystallized fruit was of course "sale" work, but a woman engaged in such work would never be confused with a shopgirl. The same magazine took note of the encouraging experience of a young cooking teacher who had been invited to live with a family for a short time while giving lessons to their cook. The woman was hesitant, fearing that the family would not appreciate the dignity of her profession and treat her as if she herself were nothing more than a cook. But she need not have worried. The family recognized "that she was a lady of cultivation and refinement, that her acquirements and ability were of a high order, and that she was entitled, therefore, to the same respect and consideration that would be accorded to a teacher of chemistry, for example." After instructing the family cook each day, the teacher was treated as if she were a guest in the house, sharing "cosy hours" with her hostess and discussing "the scientific aspects of cooking" with her host.

Whenever a domestic scientist wanted to emphasize the feminine side of the profession, the adjective "dainty" appeared. "Dainty" stood for many of the most reassuring qualities of womanhood; it was also used to temper any implication of drudgery and to give housework an important boost upward in the social scale. The year two Smith graduates opened a laundry in Brookline, Massachusetts, the write-up in *New England Kitchen Magazine* made it plain that their patrons would be "generally wealthy families, who can afford to have dainty articles daintily done." *Household News* greeted the opening of a food exposition in the nation's capital by noting that "Washington's daintiest people" had turned out for the occasion, and the manufacturers of new brands of gelatin, junket, tapioca, and cornstarch invariably featured "dainty desserts" in their advertising copy. The editor of *Household News* set a possible record for the use of the word in April 1894, when she employed it six times in three pages, mentioning among other spring menu suggestions dainty broiled sweetbreads, a dainty asparagus salad, and Indian Curry of Rice—"a dainty dish, fit for the gods."

This arduous commitment to an impossible balance between sex roles often tumbled the domestic scientists into a peculiar nether region of their own creation, where technology was as ladylike as teatime, chemistry courses trailed pleasantly into asparagus salads, and feminism was viewed as a good but dated cause. Ellen Richards would not even join the Board of Lady Managers, which was organizing the Woman's Building at the 1893 Chicago World's Fair, because she felt so strongly that women had gained all the rights of men by that time and deserved to be classed with them. "Twenty years ago I was glad to work on Woman's Boards for the education of women," she wrote to the Lady Managers. "The time is some years past when it seemed to me wise to work that way. Women have now more rights and duties than they are fitted to perform. They need to measure themselves with men on the same terms and in the same work in order to learn their own needs. Therefore the establishment of a separate woman's branch of our exposition seemed always a mistake to me. . . ." The same point was made even more strongly in a speech by the domestic expert and cookbook author Marion Harland. "Woman—with a capital letter—should by now have ceased to be a specialty," she declared. "There should be no more need of 'movements' in her behalf, and agitations for her advancement and development . . . than for the abolition of negro slavery in the United States."

In truth, while educational opportunities for women had increased greatly since the Civil War and a handful of females had managed to break into most of the traditionally male professions, these achievements had only inspired Americans of both sexes to feel complacent about the remarkable emancipation enjoyed by the ladies of the world's most enlightened nation. American women still possessed almost none of the legal rights promised by democracy, as workers or as wives or as independent adults. The feminist attack on this political distortion had been under way since early in the century, but as a consequence there was widespread feeling even among women that their problems must be over. Domestic scientists saw their revolution beginning where feminism left off, and bringing about far more dramatic changes. While feminists generally called attention to the superiority of women over men, domestic scientists thought there was room for improvement. They castigated women for being irrational, narrow-minded, and mired in the past. While feminists believed that men were blocking the way to women's fulfillment, domestic scientists believed that men were lighting the way—they had already eased the burden of housework by bestowing technology upon it, for which women seemed largely ungrateful. And while feminists fought for a share of men's privileges, a place in man's world, domestic scientists worked to create a parallel set of privileges and a female world that would mirror man's.

These visionary housekeepers modeled their activism less on the campaign for women's rights than on the dozens of social reform movements springing up around them. Many women plunged into good causes in this era, and dedicated themselves to redeeming prostitutes, improving municipal sanitation, abolishing saloons, building playgrounds for slum children, and fighting political corruption. The guiding motif for much of this work was articulated in 1888 by Frances Willard, who founded one of the first and most powerful women's reform organizations, the Woman's Christian Temperance Union. "If I were asked the mission of the ideal woman, I would reply: IT IS TO MAKE THE WHOLE WORLD HOMELIKE," she wrote. The moral and domestic virtues long associated with femininity would set the whole human family aglow, according to Frances Willard, if women would extend their influence from the private home to the public realm. Agitating for sewers and street cleaning, these reformers liked to remark, was not so very different from making sure one's own kitchen floor was clean. The domestic scientists were thoroughly in favor of what was called "municipal housekeeping," and borrowed many of its goals and methods; but here, too, they took a stance at odds with their fellow activists and distinctly their own. To make the whole world homelike would have been a major step backward, as far as they were concerned. Their own mission was to make the whole world businesslike, and the place to begin was home.

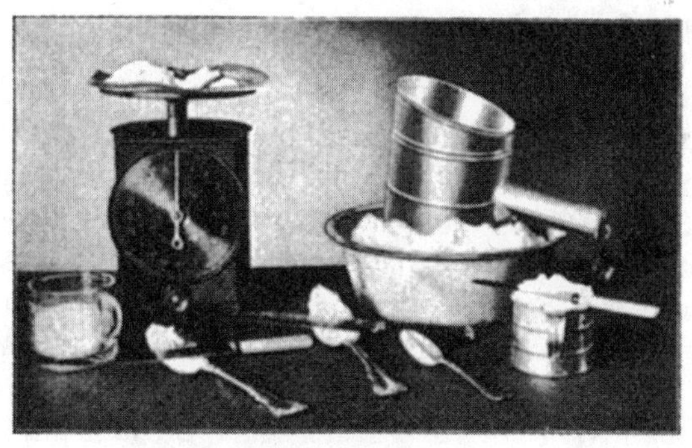

Three
Better Ways, Lighter Burdens, More Wholesome Results

While all the tasks of the household came within the scope of the domestic-science movement, it was cookery—scientific cookery—that attracted the most attention, especially as it was preached and practiced at the Boston Cooking School. The intellectual approach to the kitchen, which was the pride of the Boston Cooking School, offered women a chance to push aside some of the traditional constrictions upon their sex and stretch their minds, but in a polite way. With its borders certain and secure, scientific cookery presented a field of moral activism less daunting than many of the other popular crusades of the reform era, yet with tantalizing links to the male worlds of research, technology, business, and higher education. The women who attended the Boston Cooking School, and the careers that were born there, thrived on these links to the legitimate, the purposeful, and the rational. The meals that emerged from their preoccupations had little to do with the usual culinary concerns of appetite and enjoyment, for the messy and pedestrian task of handling food was relegated to a remote corner of the school's curriculum. These newly educated cooks pursued the science of food, not the sensuality, and worked to establish a cuisine that would be nobler, somehow, than the act of eating. "Better ways, lighter burdens, more wholesome results" was the motto of the Boston Cooking School, and during the years it presided over the American kitchen, the nation's eating habits underwent their most definitive turn toward modernity. The nation's cooks did, too, but neither of these changes took quite the form that domestic scientists had planned.

The Boston Cooking School was founded in 1879, a time when the national zeal for social progress and moral reform was rampant. Reformers of every sort had always found Boston a most congenial place in which to ply their theories, and for generations of women, Boston had long been a city receptive to projects representing the various stages of American feminism. The daringly well-educated ladies of Boston were famous throughout the nineteenth century, especially those who set themselves with vigor to the righting of wrongs. " 'She would reform the solar system if she could get hold of it,' " was Henry James's ungenerous characterization of a typical lady malcontent in *The Bostonians*. It was the Woman's Education Association, an ambitious organization powered by some of the city's most energetic female philanthropists and reformers, that came up with the idea for a cooking school. Theirs did not have the distinction of being the first cooking school in the country—the New York Cooking School had opened three years earlier—but it very quickly gained a national reputation, in part because any teaching institution located in Boston won a certain credibility from the address alone, and possibly because its founders publicized out of all proportion a rather tangential connection with Maria Parloa, the personable author of *The Appledore Cookbook*, who had recently given a popular series of cooking classes in Boston. Within two years of the school's opening, the members of the Woman's Education Association were congratulating themselves on the number of applications that had arrived from all parts of the country, and on the invitations that had been received for cooking-school graduates to open similar schools in other cities. "The wide-spread interest thus shown in the scientific cooking proves the need of the enterprise," the WEA recording secretary noted with satisfaction in the annual report.

The Woman's Education Association was already busy amassing a considerable record of accomplishments when it sent out printed leaflets announcing the Boston Cooking School. One of the association's first projects was to set up the Harvard Examinations for Women, a program that enabled women to take the entrance examinations for Harvard. Those who passed were permitted to take Harvard courses in separate, women's classes. The success of the women who took the examinations spurred the creation of the Harvard Annex, a women's branch of the university, and finally jarred the university into establishing Radcliffe College, for fear that women were about to seep into Harvard itself. The WEA had a similar effect upon the Massachusetts Institute of Technology when, with the help of Ellen Richards, it set up a women's chemistry laboratory as an annex, and eventually funded its incorporation into the school. On a more informal basis, but with equal success, the association organized outdoor botany classes for mothers, so that women might be able to enrich their children's summer vacations with botany talks and walks. A Harvard professor was in charge, and ninety women—all of them eager to exercise their minds, and reassured to know that it would make them better mothers—showed up for the first course of ten lessons.

Projects like these, which were devoted to the life of the mind, had always flourished comfortably among Bostonians, but few cities in that era would have seemed less likely to sponsor a renaissance in cooking. Boston had long treasured its Yankee reputation for plain living and high thinking; in fact, it used to vie with Cambridge, its neighbor across the Charles River, for the distinction of being the city that most ardently disdained food. According to the records of a Cambridge women's club, Cambridge society could boast a "higher tone" than Boston's, partly on account of the "simpler suppers" enjoyed by Cantabrigians. One member praised the truly stellar simplicity of the food at a reception attended by several "Cambridge notabilities": the meal consisted of bouillon, tea, and candy. Nonetheless, dinner parties in Boston could easily rival those in Cambridge for lack of festivity. One observer described the usual evening of Boston hospitality as consisting of a dinner with company you were certain to dislike, followed by a drive through Mount Auburn Cemetery, the region's most aristocratic burial ground. "Your memory of the dinner," he concluded, "is expected to reconcile you to the prospect of the graveyard." Many admirers of the Woman's Education Association must have been alarmed to see the members turn their attention to a cooking school, but the new project did not by any means represent a sudden dive toward gluttony. It was hardly the prospect of cakes and gravies for their own sake that aroused the members of the association, but rather a conviction that a cooking school could be a force for social betterment. The dismal state of America's kitchens—*Popular Science Monthly* called them "fortified intrenchments of ignorance, prejudice, irrational habits, rule of thumb, and mental vacuity"—struck them as scandalous; and they believed that educated women were the natural leaders of a domestic revolution that was only waiting to be ignited. It was time at last for sobriety, training, and reason to become the universal standards of domestic work. "In our larger towns and cities, women are saying their say on almost every topic save that of good housekeeping," pointed out a Boston leader of the YWCA. "There are many women who make their homes a paradise of rest and comfort, but their voices are not heard in the land; if a good apostle of homes came among them, they would rally to her support, I think." The WEA hoped that its cooking school would act as that good apostle, attracting support and emulation throughout the country.

As a plan for instruction in practical matters, rather than Latin or botany, the cooking-school idea did differ from some of the WEA's other projects. But its emphasis on useful skills reflected an attitude toward reform that had been gaining in popularity among progressive philanthropists ever since the social and economic upheavals of industrialization brought wave after wave of poverty and distress to their attention. Dispensing charity at random seemed futile to these purposeful benefactors: they wanted to go more directly to the roots of unemployment and depravity by teaching children to develop dexterity and good work habits. Manual training for boys and sewing for girls were introduced into the Boston public schools at mid-century, and the trend spread to other cities during the next decades. Training the hand as well as the mind was important in every social class, these reformers often claimed, and they liked to think that by instituting such training on a democratic basis they were engendering new respect for the lowly occupations of housework and manual labor.

Philanthropy in this key was much on the minds of the women who organized the Woman's Education Association, and its standing committees from the very start included a Committee on Industrial Education. The idea of opening a cooking school occurred to the ladies of the Industrial Committee, as they referred to themselves, early on, but the minutes of their meetings reveal considerable uncertainty and a great deal of floundering. The pristine task of sewing was easy enough to embrace, but the prospect of cookery raised some discomfiting questions. "While this Committee regret that they have done nothing directly in the way of Industrial Education, they have not been idle," a member assured the WEA when she offered the Industrial Committee's annual report for 1873. She went on to explain that the committee had spent "nearly all the winter" investigating the ways and means of establishing a cooking school but had been unable to come up with a plan. The chief problem, with which they were still grappling, was what to do with all the food that would be prepared. The committee had not yet been able to come up with a way to make use of the soups and roasts and loaves that would be the unavoidable result of such an undertaking. They held discussions for a time with the School of Technology in hopes that the new technology building would house a refectory of some sort, which might be linked with their cooking school and so "afford the indispensable opportunity of disposing of the food when cooked," but the effort at collaboration did not work out. For the time being, the committee had given up the whole idea.

Evidently there was never any suggestion during these discussions that the cooking students themselves might eat the food. This omission was one of the first signs of a persistent, irreconcilable standoff between the functions of cooking and eating that would characterize scientific cookery for decades. By contrast the committee had no trouble organizing a much less ambiguous culinary reform, which one of the members had observed in operation in New York. This was a diet kitchen, set up in conjunction with a hospital to supply food to needy patients. The committee launched a similar enterprise at the New England Hospital for Women and Children, where at little or no cost a patient could obtain food tickets from her doctor and redeem them at the diet kitchen for the appropriate gruels, jellies, and milk soups. The life-sustaining function of food was never difficult for the committee to respect, but they struggled hard over what appeared to be purely gratuitous aspects of eating.

Not until the New York Cooking School began making a name for itself several years later did the Industrial Committee return to its original project. In New York a charitable organization much like the WEA had been offering cooking lessons to working-class girls and women, as well as lessons in more elaborate cookery for ladies, and the publicity was considerable. There is no indication in the minutes that anyone from the Industrial Committee visited the New York Cooking School, but it seems likely; for after their first impulse had lain dormant for five years, the members suddenly bestirred themselves in February 1879 and began to appoint subcommittees.

Their initial plan was to hire the renowned Maria Parloa to instruct a normal, or teacher-training, class for three months that spring, thus creating a faculty for a school on a larger scale that could open in the fall. A suite of rooms at 158 Tremont Street was donated, a subcommittee went to work on the still-troublesome issue of "distribution of food," and other members set about raising money and gathering the necessary supplies. Almost immediately the subcommittee that had been sent to interview Miss Parloa returned with a discouraging report: she was charging twenty dollars for two lessons, more than they could afford if the cost to pupils was to be kept as low as possible. At a time when many women teaching in city schools earned perhaps ten dollars a week, while male schoolteachers made nearly three times that amount, Miss Parloa's fee represented a remarkable income for a woman. She had been teaching and lecturing in the Boston area for only two years, but was greatly in demand and appears to have been a formidable businesswoman. One member of the Industrial Committee knew of another candidate, however: Joanna Sweeney, a young woman who had been running her own small, private classes in cookery for six years, and could bring her own equipment. Joanna—she was the only woman who appeared in the records of the WEA under her first name, without the dignity of "Miss"—was not at all the sort of lady the committee had in mind to personify the Boston Cooking School, for she was an obscure Irish cooking teacher without standing or reputation. They finally agreed to use her temporarily and hired her for one month, at the rate of two dollars per lesson, appointing a committee member to monitor the lessons each day. They also secured Miss Parloa to give public lecture-demonstrations every other Saturday. When the circulars announcing the opening of the Boston Cooking School came out, the instructors were advertised as Miss Parloa and a "competent teacher."

The school was organized in some haste, and on a tiny start-up budget. The WEA managed to channel $100 their way, and a few small contributions came in from individual members and their friends. Only the newly revived enthusiasm of the committee members made it possible for them to open the school just four weeks after voting to go ahead with the idea. The subcommittee on supplies obtained most of them from one another: Mrs. Foster gave towels, Mrs. Thomas hemmed them; Mrs. Towne gave a lock, a broom, and some dishpans; Mrs. Hooper gave spoons and soap. Several ladies were eager to lecture on cookery themselves, offering to show up on short notice whenever needed; these offers were graciously recorded. The subcommittee on pupils canvassed the public schools and local parishes and missions, writing personal notes of inquiry to a number of ministers, and two ladies prepared "advertisements and editorials" for the Boston newspapers. It was decided to charge a dollar and a half for a course of six lessons designed for "daughters of mechanics." These would be the girls and women of families with an income of about $350 to $500 a year. The fee was low enough for the ladies of the committee to assume that even in families where the equivalent of a day's wages might have to be sacrificed, the economical ways in cookery that the pupils would bring home would in short time pay for the lessons. Classes for privately employed cooks, however, would be a dollar apiece, since the mistress of the household would be paying for them. Admission to Miss Parloa's demonstration lessons would be fifty cents for ladies and half price for public-school girls. A committee member would keep track of the pupils and payments each day, making sure to record names, addresses, and "descriptions" of the pupils accurately. This was deemed necessary because students who completed a course of lessons were to be given certificates, which they could present as references in applying for positions as domestic cooks, and the committee was anxious to avoid misuse of the certificates. Finally, less than twenty-four hours before the Boston Cooking School opened its doors, the Industrial Committee decided that food cooked during the lessons "should be given to needy pupils."

According to respectful news stories printed in the *Boston Transcript* and the *Boston Advertiser*, seven pupils were waiting on the doorstep when the cooking school opened on March 10, 1879, at nine in the morning. The girls were not identified, although the *Advertiser* commented approvingly that all of them planned to become "practical housekeepers." It seems most probable that the seven were, if not precisely the mechanics' daughters for whom the fees had been set, young women of equally humble expectations who would be keeping house on a small budget for their parents or husbands.

The committee was hoping to attract another important constituency as well: potential cooks and servants for private homes, and employed cooks who wanted to improve their skills. A great deal of the public interest in the cooking school, and the financial support that was culled from friends and well-wishers, undoubtedly reflected the rising despair among more affluent ladies about how to staff their households. Only a small percentage of American homes employed help, but they included the homes of many of the most prominent female writers and activists, and these women were creating a tremendous cottage industry in theoretical solutions to the servant problem. Training working-class girls for domestic service was an obvious priority for the Boston Cooking School at its inception; nonetheless, as the *Transcript* pointed out reassuringly, "Some ladies who do not keep servants are anxious to be admitted . . . so that the classes will by no means be made up exclusively of servants, or of young girls anxious to go into service."

The lesson for the first day had been planned and voted on by the Industrial Committee, who plainly had in mind the kitchens of working-class Boston. Tomato soup, Irish stew with mutton and potatoes, and steamed apple pudding were on the menu, and the students also mixed bread dough, which the next day's class would make into loaves and rolls. Each student had a notebook, an apron, and a hand towel, and they took turns mixing and measuring under Joanna Sweeney's direction. Evidently they were all adjudged "needy," for at the end of the lesson the whole class sat down to dine. The following Saturday Miss Parloa gave her first demonstration, which appears to have been highly successful, certainly among the ladies of the Industrial Committee, who promptly voted to admit themselves to her future lessons at half price. (Another audience member well satisfied with Miss Parloa's demonstration was the prominent philanthropist Mary Hemenway, who purchased for three dollars all the food prepared at the demonstration and carried it home for lunch.) With alacrity the committee decided to take responsibility for planning Miss Parloa's menus as well as Joanna's, and they showed no interest in Irish stew and apple pudding. Miss Parloa's next Saturday demonstration was a lavish entertainment featuring larded grouse with bread sauce, lobster croquettes, potato soufflé, cream meringues, and orange sherbet. At the beginning of the second week of school, so many ladies had inquired about lessons—ladies, it was stressed in the committee's minutes, "who wish to make direct use of instruction in cooking"—that the committee decided to establish special Wednesday and Saturday classes for them, charging three dollars for six lessons, or twice what the mechanics' daughters paid.

Despite all this excitement about the school, or perhaps because of it, the subcommittee on Disposal of Food was still sifting through possible solutions to their dilemma. Permitting the students to eat what they had cooked certainly disposed of the food, but to what end? The committee could see no lasting benefit in this solution in terms of either charity or economy. At one point they thought of sending out the cooked food to poor people; then they discarded that idea in favor of having poor people come to the school to get it. Tentatively they concluded that the food should be sold at cost "to such poor people as would come for it, bringing their own baskets and kettles, and to such of the scholars as wished to buy it." A price sheet was drawn up, listing the usual dishes prepared in class—chiefly soups, pork and beans, bread, croquettes, and gingerbread—at prices ranging from ten cents for a small sheet of gingerbread to a dollar for a dozen fish balls. This experiment came close enough to recouping the cost of the food to inspire the committee to rule that each class, after its first lesson, "should be restricted to merely tasting the food, not wholly consuming it." A complementary ruling followed immediately—that the same spoon should never be used twice for tasting without being washed.

The immediate and enthusiastic public response to

the Boston Cooking School during its first three-month term that spring seemed to make it imperative that the school reopen in the fall, but when September arrived the committee—which now called itself the Cooking School Committee—was faced with a new set of concerns. They strongly felt the need to hire a more seemly teacher than Joanna Sweeney, the donor of the rooms at 158 Tremont Street was charging rent now, and they wanted to reorganize the school so that they might offer different courses at different prices to ladies, working-class girls, and would-be cooking teachers. Replacing Joanna Sweeney was the most difficult problem, and after a fruitless search they agreed in desperation to take on the sister of a friend of one of the committee members. Mary J. Lincoln was virtually without professional experience as either a cook or a teacher, but the women who interviewed her must have seen something of her potential, for she went on to become one of the best-known cooks of her generation and indeed something of a cult figure, at least in the pages of the journal she helped found and edit, *New England Kitchen Magazine*. In an early issue of *New England Kitchen*, Mrs. Lincoln told the story of how she began her career, suddenly forced to earn a living on account of financial "reverses" suffered by her husband and his consequent ill health. After taking a few odd jobs in sewing and cleaning, she wrote, she was persuaded to accept the position of principal at the Boston Cooking School, where she started out armed with nothing but her own experience as a housekeeper, a few lessons "in fancy dishes" from Joanna Sweeney, and attendance at a single demonstration lesson by Miss Parloa. "This gave me a clear conception of the work to be done," she stated. "The ignorance shown by some of my pupils increased my confidence in my own knowledge. . . . My work for the next five years at the cooking school speaks for itself."

For the most part Mrs. Lincoln's highly successful career does speak for itself, but this account of her apprenticeship contained a little judicious skimming. According to the terms of her initial agreement with the Cooking School Committee, she was hired on the condition that she first take two full weeks of lessons with Joanna Sweeney and Miss Parloa, tuition and carfare paid by the committee, after which she would teach for a month on approval. Her salary would be $75 a month, slightly less than what Joanna Sweeney was making. Her first month of teaching was acceptable enough for her to be retained for the winter —in fact, she and Mr. Lincoln moved into two spare rooms at the school and set up housekeeping there—but as the term went on, the committee spent several meetings arguing about her. Evidently a number of students expressed dissatisfaction with Mrs. Lincoln's teaching, and the committee, still hoping that Miss Parloa might be persuaded to take over the school, sent a few members on a furtive mission to query her about possibly replacing Mrs. Lincoln. This group reported that Miss Parloa would only accept the position if the school was expanded considerably and moved into grander quarters. Unfortunately, even the exceedingly casual records kept by the school treasurer showed a sizable deficit, which had appeared as soon as the school began paying rent and was getting larger every month. With reluctance the committee set aside the idea of expansion for the time being. Miss Parloa agreed to take on a normal class twice a week, and in response to the continuing protests against Mrs. Lincoln, the committee decided she should be enrolled in the normal class herself. After a few months with Miss Parloa on the payroll, however—she had raised her fee to $25 a lesson—the committee had accumulated such a large debt to her that it was thought wisest to let her go and to have the freshly trained Mrs. Lincoln teach the course. This caused such an uproar among the normal students that the committee hastily rehired Miss Parloa for one class a week. In the meantime the committee had to prepare its annual report on the cooking school to the main body of the WEA. "The Committee feel that they have every reason to congratulate themselves on having Mrs. Lincoln at the head of the school," the chairwoman told the WEA smoothly; ". . . her many qualities as a woman make her influence upon the School particularly valuable."

Two years after its opening, then, the Boston Cooking School had become an active and well-known institution that was overwhelmingly in debt. Miss Parloa was draining the treasury as fast as she attracted pupils, and as the school expanded it continually needed more equipment and supplies. Several gentlemen had been invited to join the committee when the need for fund-raising became serious, and with their financial connections a few subscriptions and donations were attracted. Apart from its financial problems the school was thriving: between the winters of 1881 and 1882 the number of pupils nearly doubled, to approximately four hundred. After her uncertain start Mrs. Lincoln rapidly developed into a popular teacher—soon, in fact, she was being sought out as a guest lecturer, and on her very first speaking engagement, in Southboro, Massachusetts, she was able to command a $25 fee, the equal of Miss Parloa's. Over a thousand women flocked to her public demonstrations during the winter of 1882, and graduates of the normal class were finding employment all over the country. It became apparent to the committee that the school was doing too well to close, while the debt was too frightening to ignore; consequently they voted to disengage the school from the Woman's Education Association and incorporate it as a separate body. "Henceforth," scribbled the secretary in her minutes, "all arrangements must be made in a business like manner."

Perhaps the most businesslike step taken by the new corporation was to acknowledge the fact that the Boston Cooking School could no longer claim to be a charitable enterprise. "The attempt to make it altogether self-supporting, or to confine it to the poorer classes, have both been abandoned," admitted Mrs. Hooper, a committee member now president of the new corporation, in her first annual report. The Woman's Education Association made much the same point in its own report summing up the work of the cooking school as it separated from its parent organization. "The original purpose was purely a charitable one, and the field of operation was intended to be among the poorest classes," explained the WEA. "But ample means alone could secure the working out of this plan." According to both accounts, the school simply could not pay for itself with the low rates it was charging, or command much in the way of donations. Evidently the founders hoped that, by incorporating, the school would be able to establish an endowment and then perhaps support work of a wider beneficence. For the moment, however, the Boston Cooking School was to retreat from philanthropy and take up the pleasant business of serving its most prominent constituency—what the WEA called a "class of housekeepers who could afford to pay for their lessons." After all, noted Mrs. Hooper in her report, ". . . that a woman is rich seems no sufficient reason for excluding her from the advantages offered her of becoming practically conversant with some of the most important duties of woman's home life."

To be sure, a certain measure of their obligation to the poor had been taken care of ever since the winter of 1880, when the ladies in charge of the cooking school had been offered the sum of one hundred dollars by another charitable group to establish free cooking classes for poor women. The Cooking School Committee debated at some length whether to use the money to pay tuition for thirty-three women, who would be sent from Boston's Italian district to take classes at the cooking school, or to open a branch of the school right in the district itself. All but one of the committee members felt the poor would benefit most by traveling to Tremont Street, but that one member—author and educator Lucretia P. Hale—argued so strongly for opening a branch in the Italian neighborhood that the vote was turned around in her favor. Miss Hale was right, of course. Very few lower-class women ever found their way to the Boston Cooking School, but its North Bennett Street branch flourished from the start. The kitchen and dining room of an old sailors' home were rented, and classes were scheduled for three evenings a week and Saturdays. As many as ninety-six girls at a time attended the Saturday classes, and over two hundred women frequently turned out for the evening lectures. Miss Parloa was hired to give a few of the lectures—but only a few, since she demanded her standard fee even from worthy causes—and additional teachers had to be selected according to more modest requirements. Several ladies from the Cooking School Committee volunteered, and the undemanding Joanna Sweeney was called upon once again. The North Bennett Street school was meant to remain open only as long as the original hundred dollars held out, but expenses were so low that the school managed to continue for several years.

After its charitable work, the Boston Cooking School took most seriously its effort to train cooks for domestic service, but here, too, the corporation's first annual report is touched with a sense of regret. When the school first opened, lessons for cooks had been offered at a dollar apiece, on the assumption that mistresses would pay gladly to improve the cooking in their own homes. Perhaps they would have, but very few mistresses were willing to free their cooks from the kitchen in order for them to attend classes, and not many cooks could be persuaded to come on their afternoons off. The committee had somewhat better luck instituting a series of evening lectures for cooks, at twenty-five cents each, but the school couldn't afford to maintain such an inexpensive series, and the response from local domestics was still discouraging. At the same time the plea for good help was louder than ever, and the cry constantly heard from the community was, as the report put it, "Why does not the School give us more experienced cooks as the practical result of all this instruction?" In the face of this pressure the school set up a special fund to accept donations in support of lessons for cooks. According to the corporation secretary, who included a statement in the first annual report, contributions to this Housekeepers' Fund were coming in at a rate "slower . . . than had been anticipated," and according to the president, the number of servants applying "has been smaller than was anticipated." Nevertheless, both officers expressed the belief that the cooking school would accomplish a great deal of good in this area, very soon. The WEA was less optimistic. "Cooks will not spend time and money for a training which is not required, and from which they can expect no immediate practical advantage," its report concluded. Eventually the Boston Cooking School gave up the struggle to create an improved servant class, but many members of the WEA persisted as hopefully as ever. Twenty years later a WEA committee was busy setting up a fanciful employment project called the Household Aid Company—"a much-to-be-desired elevation in the dignity of household work"—which lasted only a little longer than the one-dollar lessons for cooks instituted a generation earlier.

Once the ladies in charge of the Boston Cooking School had accepted the fact that they could not afford to put too much emphasis on helping the poor, and that training domestic servants was largely a thankless task, they willingly turned their attention to the instruction of women very much like themselves. "Ladies' Practice Classes" became an important feature of the curriculum and were established on three levels: Plain Cooking, Richer Cooking, and Fancy Cooking. In setting up these three courses Mrs. Lincoln chose a considerably more democratic method than was displayed at the New York Cooking School, where practice classes reflected distinct social as well as culinary goals. The New York school offered four courses: the First Artisan Course ("for the instruction of the young daughters of working people"), the Second Artisan Course ("for the grown daughters and wives of workingmen"), the Plain Cooks' Course ("for young housewives beginning married life in comfortable or moderate circumstances"), and the Ladies' Course in Middle Class and Artistic Cookery. The particular dishes assigned to each level of study carefully matched these shades of meaning: when preparing fish, for example, the First Artisans made boiled haddock with parsley sauce; the Second Artisans fixed boiled ray with piquante sauce; the Plain Cooks made boiled cod with hollandaise sauce; and the Ladies worked on halibut filets *à la Maréchale*.

The allocation of dishes at the Boston Cooking School was along comparable lines but on a far more relaxed basis. In time Mrs. Lincoln learned the niceties of refined and decorative cookery, but she had been raised on what could only be called plain food—especially the characteristically New England dishes like baked beans, brown bread, fish balls, doughnuts, and Indian pudding—and these remained the anchor of her cuisine. More adamantly scientific cooks would have cringed to see heavy, humble doughnuts on an educated lady's menu, but Mrs. Lincoln's approach to food was not very dogmatic—a scientific theory followed by a piece of blueberry pie was approximately her style. While French cooking, or at least French terminology, was coming into vogue for upper-class dining, Mrs. Lincoln generally taught the dishes she knew best. In all three courses at the cooking school she concentrated on standard American preparations and tried to avoid using French terms, so that her highest course in Fancy Cooking dwelt on fried fish, fried celery, floating island, and pigs-in-blankets—not a great deal more exotic than the food in Richer Cooking (flannel cakes, apple pie, and Turkish pilaf) or even Plain Cooking (which culminated in potato puff, plain lobster, and French dressing). Unlike some of her conscientiously abstemious colleagues, Mrs. Lincoln openly appreciated a good dessert, French or not, and a sweet concluded every lesson in every course, with the occasional exception of breakfast. Halfway through Richer Cooking, and again halfway through Fancy Cooking, the lessons would begin to include from two to five desserts. Mrs. Lincoln sent home her Fancy Cooking students after a final banquet that was lavish if not exactly balanced: sweetbreads prepared four different ways, and a string of desserts including Strawberry Charlotte, Frozen Pudding, Café Parfait, and *Gâteau de Princess Louise.*

While these courses in cookery for ladies attracted popular attention to the Boston Cooking School, the founders and teachers were proudest of their more elevated branches of instruction. After their success in establishing the diet kitchen at the New England Hospital for Women and Children, the committee made sure to include Invalid Cookery in the public demonstration lessons from the very beginning. The Boston Cooking School quickly earned a reputation for its lessons in sickroom cookery, for most sick people were tended at home and it was the women of the family who were called upon to do the nursing. The relationship between diet and healing was clear to scientific cooks, although non-specific, and in the attention they paid to sickroom cookery they were far ahead of most members of the medical profession in their time or ours. The students in both Plain and Richer Cooking devoted time to foods suitable for invalids—beef tea, Irish-moss lemonade, tapioca, and lemon or wine jelly—and the school also offered a special Nurses' Course for women who were interested in the still new notion of professional training for nurses. In these twelve lessons the nursing students made dozens of varieties of gruels, mushes, jellies, and custards, as well as some roasted and broiled meats and a score of strengthening desserts. The entire span of an illness was taken into account, from the early stages when a patient could manage only beef tea and flour gruel, to the days, presumably approaching complete recovery, when venison and charlotte russe were called for. After the cooking school had been in operation for only three seasons, the founders were greatly pleased to receive a letter from Dr. Minot of the Harvard Medical School asking if classes in sickroom cookery could be arranged for medical students. They could indeed—the Boston Cooking School's association with the Harvard Medical School went on for many years and remained one of the cooking school's most treasured distinctions.

The work for which the cooking school was most widely respected, however, and the work that came first in the sentiments of its founders and teachers, was the training of the normal class. Graduates of the Boston Cooking School had been in demand ever since the pupils in Miss Parloa's first normal classes completed their study and went right out to teach in the public schools and to give cooking classes in other cities. During the 1880s and 1890s, women who trained at cooking schools found a growing number of professions opening up: they could take charge of school and hospital kitchens, become the matrons at prisons and asylums, run tearooms or small catering services, give public lectures on cookery and diet, create recipes and demonstrate new products for food manufacturers, and of course teach cooking—to children, to working girls, to slum dwellers, to ladies, to immigrants, and even to men. There was an urgent need, as the Boston Cooking School's first annual report said strongly, for cooking teachers "to lift this great social incubus of bad cooking and its incident evils from the households of the country at large." The course of study for normal pupils at the Boston Cooking School, after the first uneasy months in which teaching responsibilities flipped back and forth between Miss Parloa and Mrs. Lincoln, settled into a sober curriculum in which cookery itself played a relatively small part. At the height of the school's reputation in the 1890s the course ran for six months and included Psychology, Physiology and Hygiene, Bacteriology, Foods, Laundry Work, and the Chemistry of Soap, Bluing, and Starch. Three different classes in cooking were required, although two of them—Cookery Applied to Public School Work, and Observation and Assistance at Public Schools—focused more on teaching than on food preparation. Cooking—that is, the actual mixing, measuring, boiling, and baking—was taught under the heading Laboratory Practice. An elective in Household Sanitation was offered, examinations were held in all required courses, and the school year culminated each June with full-scale commencement exercises.

This comprehensive curriculum was designed above all else for preparedness. If a cooking student from a modest financial background was fortunate enough to marry into grander circumstances, she would be perfectly equipped to take charge of a new household, however large and complicated. If, conversely, an affluent graduate found herself plunged into poverty—the way Mrs. Lincoln did when her husband suffered "reverses"—she would be able to earn a respectable living. When a young woman received her diploma from the Boston Cooking School she was receiving accreditation for a future that seemed, perhaps for the first time, under control. And this pursuit of control extended all the way through her training, until every potential domestic crisis had been accounted for and every detail of the kitchen had been magnified for inspection and analysis. An education at the Boston Cooking School was an education in womanhood itself, womanhood at its most modern, womanhood with a touch of the intellectual about it. Every graduate stepped into the world as a lady and a scholar, taking equal pride in both facets of her achievement. "The demand is that the girl shall not only practice cooking, sewing and cleaning, for example, but that she shall be trained to think," a cooking teacher emphasized. "To think about cooking and sewing and cleaning, if you please, and to think exactly, logically, and to a purpose." The kind of thinking taught at the Boston Cooking School was displayed to the public once a year during the school's commencement exercises, which featured—in lieu of valedictory addresses—miniature lecture-demonstrations by the most talented graduates.

The ceremonies honoring the class of 1897 were typical: they were held in the school's largest lecture hall, draped for the occasion in green and white, the school colors. The same color scheme was carried out in the refreshments, which included green-and-white olive sandwiches, green-and-white frosted cakes, and green-and-white bonbons. Alumnae, friends and family of the graduating class, trustees, and some visiting teachers from other schools made up the audience, and after the usual welcoming speeches, the first graduate, Hannah W. Haines of Passaic, New Jersey, stepped to the worktable. Miss Haines's topic was "Fuel and Combustion" and she began with experiments showing the effect of air on combustion, using a candle and a glass tube. She then turned to a model stove perched on the worktable, and built a little fire. Alice Chamberlain of St. Louis, Missouri, spoke next on "Eggs," holding up and describing one egg after another, from the tiny hummingbird egg to the large goose egg. She made the point that all eggs were edible, including crocodile eggs, and prepared an omelet soufflé in a chafing dish. A presentation on "The American Lobster" was made by Emily Tillinghast of Worcester, Massachusetts, who displayed a lobster—for demonstration purposes she substituted a three-inch crawfish—and killed it in boiling water, noting the change of color from green to red. Then she took up a real lobster, killed previously, and dissected it, calling attention to each part of its anatomy. The lobster meat was put to use in the next demonstration, by Ada D. Wagg of Lisbon, Maine, who made "Hawaiian Curry" according to a recipe sent to one of the graduates by a relative in Hawaii. Finally, Alice Bradley of Hyde Park, Massachusetts, spoke on a new method of instruction called "Individual Work." In teaching cookery, Miss Bradley told her audience, the instructor should divide the recipe so that each student uses just enough ingredients to make a single portion. In that way the student learns the process from beginning to end and can compare results usefully with her classmates, rather than simply taking a turn occasionally in the lesson. Miss Bradley demonstrated by making a single portion of strawberry shortcake.

Commencement morning itself was not long enough to include any but these fairly quick presentations, so during the final weeks of school a special series of public demonstrations was held in order to allow ambitious students to show off the kind of work that called for more time and more elaborate equipment. In the spring of 1897, Miss Chamberlain and Miss Tillinghast were featured in this special series, and they gave a detailed presentation of a luncheon in green and white. The audience arrived to find on stage a table set with a damask cloth covered by a square of green silk, upon which was placed a bowl of lilies of the valley. Smilax and maidenhair ferns had been arranged along the edges of the table with some precision, to look as if they had been dropped there by a careless hand, and plates of green-and-white cake were set down. Breadsticks, cut three-eighths of an inch in width and thickness, had been tied in bundles of three with green ribbon and placed on the table, along with dishes of salted almonds and green bonbons. Miss Chamberlain and Miss Tillinghast had created a four-course green-and-white menu, and they prepared and discussed each dish while the audience looked on: cream of pea soup; sweetbreads sauté, with asparagus in cream sauce, and spinach in heart-shaped croustades; watercress and cucumber salad with cream dressing; and pistachio *bombe glacée aux fruits*. When everything was ready the two cooks sat down at the table and, to complete their luncheon, ate it. Two of their classmates acted as waitresses, demonstrating to the audience the correct way of serving each course. In the same series that spring, four students worked together to present a pink dinner, two more to give a red-and-white luncheon, and one—the only student to select a non-culinary topic for her demonstration—made two kinds of laundry starch and ironed a shirtwaist.

A deft hand with cream sauce and laundry starch may not seem to constitute a very revolutionary accomplishment, but the fact that a woman had gone to school to learn these skills—and not merely the skills but the abiding reasons why heat acts upon starch in such a way as to produce cream sauce—made her more of an iconoclast than she might have appeared in her cap and apron. Cooking-school graduates personified a welcome new definition of women's worth and function, a definition that was beginning to seize the imaginations of middle- and upper-class Americans with a taste for the modern, but not exactly the feminist, female. Club members, restless housekeepers, and women planning careers that could be kept under control were drawn to scientific cookery—educated cookery—in numbers that gratified the founders of the Boston Cooking School. Within the domestic-science movement, cookery had few significant rivals, for the challenges posed by plumbing, house construction, and laundry never aroused the kind of attention among women that Ellen Richards had hoped. With the exception of a few professionals drawn to architecture and cleaning solvents, most women applied their liveliest curiosity to food. In the years following the founding of the Boston Cooking School, newspapers and magazines gave ever-increasing amounts of space to recipes and cooking tips, and women of every social degree attended cooking classes at club meetings, settlement houses,

YWCAs, and an array of cooking schools. Reform groups and charitable organizations took up scientific cookery as a study topic or a new cause, and the same groups agitated successfully for children's cooking classes in the public schools.

New England Kitchen Magazine, which began publication in April 1894, regularly covered events of note in scientific cookery, and news items from its first few issues give an idea of the range of activities then under way. In the summer of that year the magazine reported on commencement exercises at three schools in Boston—the Boston Cooking School, the YWCA School of Domestic Science, and the Boston Normal School of Cookery—as well as at the New York Cooking School, the Philadelphia Cooking School, and Pratt Institute in New York (where Ellen Richards spoke to the graduating class on "The Preservation of the Home"). In Boston the Saturday Afternoon Girls' Club held its second anniversary meeting, at which over a hundred girls exhibited their work in sewing, clay modeling, wood carving, and millinery, as well as cooking. " 'I made a lamb stew for breakfast this morning,' said one girl, 'and father said 'twas very good.' " The Cooking Teachers' Club held its annual meeting, and on that occasion Fannie Farmer, appointed a year earlier as principal of the Boston Cooking School, was presented with a gift in return for hostessing many of the previous meetings and providing "some dainty refreshment" for the members. Summer cooking courses were announced, sponsored by the Chautauqua Assemblies in Long Island, Maine, Pennsylvania, and Michigan. At the main Chautauqua Assembly at Lake Chautauqua, New York, the cookery department was to be run by Emma P. Ewing, author of *Cooking and Castle-Building*, whose lessons would include Chafing Dish Cookery, Some Simple Puddings, and A Dainty Breakfast.

Reports from local cooking-school graduates who were at work in New England and elsewhere also ran in the magazine, often under the heading "Somewhat Personal," or "Personal Paragraphs." Mrs. Perry was teaching in Augusta and Portland, Maine, where special interest had been aroused by her lecture on "Cookery from an Educational Point of View." Miss Young was employed by a flour manufacturer to give demonstrations in baking bread and cake, and, having traveled through "the principal towns of Vermont," she was now baking in Pennsylvania. Miss Clarke, principal of the Milwaukee Cooking School, was lecturing in the South; and " 'What do you think I found on one of the very first trips I made in this delightful town?' " she reported from Asheville, North Carolina. " 'A cooking class in full session poring over "The Boston Cook Book." . . . Everything was excellent, with the familiar flavor that lent an extra zest.' " As a graduate of the Boston Cooking School, Miss Clarke herself had learned to cook from *Mrs. Lincoln's Boston Cook Book*, the school's main teaching text for over ten years. Another graduate, Miss Nichols, sent word that she "arranges lunch parties for ladies who have not confidence in their own ability or that of their cooks. . . ." And in Boston, up to five hundred ladies had attended each of Mrs. Lincoln's cooking demonstrations sponsored by Jordan, Marsh and Co., the department store. The series of six demonstrations had concluded with "quite an ovation."

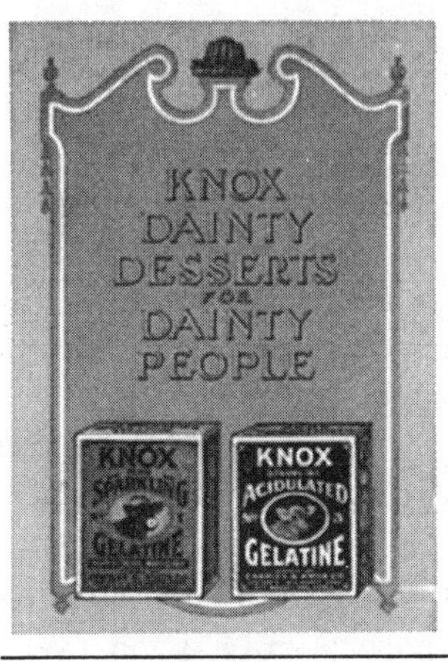

Four
Perfection Salad

Cooking magazines, cooking columns in the newspapers, cooking clubs, cooking schools, training programs for cooking teachers, cookbooks of every size and style—"Now, what does all this interest in cookery mean?" asked Mary Lincoln. She was addressing the World's Congress of Women at the Chicago World's Fair, and she went ahead and answered her own question. "We think that it means that many of our people have awakened to the fact that eating is something more than animal indulgence, and that cooking has a nobler purpose than the gratification of appetite and the sense of taste. Cooking has been defined as 'the art of preparing food for the nourishment of the human body.' "

Mrs. Lincoln's preference for this definition was shared by most of the teachers and writers who were her colleagues in scientific cookery. These were women, who, like Mrs. Lincoln, had been cooking teachers even before they were cooks, or who had prepared for the work by going to cooking school. Their culinary imaginations were organized according to categories of food value, systematic measurements, kitchen procedures, and the process of digestion. The copious recipes that emerged from cooking schools were not in themselves revolutionary, at least in the early years, for Mrs. Lincoln and the other teachers tended to rely on the familiar British-based cookery of New England, venturing occasionally into the realm of French sauces and desserts. But their beliefs about food had a greater effect on these dishes than many more imaginative cooks might have achieved. By ennobling the recipes over the results, and disdaining the proof of the palate, they made it possible for American cooking to accept a flood of damaging innovations for years to come. Cooking-school cookery emphasized every aspect of food except the notion of taste; and similarly, the only procedure of kitchen or dining room that nearly always passed without mention was the act of eating. Students at cooking schools practiced meal planning, marketing, cooking, and garnishing the dish; they learned the correct way to serve and remove each course; they might give attention to the proprieties of conversation and social atmosphere at the dining table; and they tirelessly scrutinized their food through microscopes for evidence of starch, acidity, or adulteration. But to enjoy food, to develop a sense for flavors, or to acknowledge that eating could be a pleasure in itself had virtually no part in any course, lecture, or magazine article. What Mrs. Lincoln called the "gratification of appetite" would hardly have made an honorable goal for a scientific profession, and more important, it would have invaded that certain discreet distance separating a lady from her food. Slimness and dieting did not become national passions until well into the twentieth century, but there was a long-standing assumption that well-bred women were creatures with light, disinterested eating habits. Even the heftiest of the scientific cooks made a point of impressing the public with how meagerly they ate at home ("I am afraid the majority of people would feel quite starved," confessed Sarah Tyson Rorer of the Philadelphia Cooking School, describing her weekly fare. In truth, Mrs. Rorer's solid figure attested to an excellent appetite and so, for that matter, did her home menus). Unlike earlier periods of American life, the turn of the century was a time when good health was generally admired in women, and the importance of nutrition and physical exercise was beginning to be widely recognized. Yet even in this era, too much evidence of an overt fondness for food would have made a woman appear gross and unfeminine.

"'I came home cross to-night, cross as a bear with a sore head,'" admits the husband of a young bride who is with difficulty learning to cook, in a serial that ran in *The Woman's Home Companion*. "'I have been cross all day. I thought it was business worries. I know now that I was hungry. . . . I suppose you women don't know anything about that, eh?'

"'No,' said Martha, thoughtfully. 'I doubt if we do. I have often forgotten to eat until reminded by faintness and headache that it was past dinner or luncheon time. . . .'

"'A man would have been ready to murder his brother by that time. We're built that way,'" explains her husband.

It was in the well-regulated functioning of protein, carbohydrate, and fat, and in the marvelous mechanisms of the digestive process, that scientific cooks found their culinary romance. The science of nutrition had progressed far enough by the 1890s to offer a coherent and in many ways accurate picture of the use of foods in the human body, although the blank spots in the available information prompted a rather distorted perspective, especially on the part of enthusiasts like the new professionals. Many of them based their teaching and writing on the work of W. O. Atwater, a professor of chemistry at Wesleyan University who became something of a mentor to scientific cooks. Atwater had studied in Germany, where much of the leading research in nutrition was going on, before taking up his position at Wesleyan, and he set in motion the first major American investigations into food and digestion. In studies requested variously by the Smithsonian, the Chicago World's Fair, the Department of Labor, and the U.S. Fish Commission, Atwater undertook the chemical analysis of much of the American diet, item by item. At the same time, he was promoting the establishment of state agricultural experiment stations, modeled on similar enterprises developed in Europe. Scientific research in agriculture was under way in fourteen states by the time the federal government opened an Office of Experiment Stations and put Atwater in charge of it. Later he returned to full-time teaching and research, but at his urging the mandate of the experiment stations was officially extended to include the study of human, as well as animal, nutrition. Bulletins on food and diet from the Office of Experiment Stations began to circulate throughout the country, and along with Atwater's magazine articles, they were frequently quoted in domestic-science literature. Atwater was also one of the few chemists willing to introduce women into his field. At Wesleyan and at the state experiment station in Connecticut he accepted women as special students, laboratory assistants, and researchers, and he took a gratifying interest in the domestic-science movement.

Atwater's most definitive contribution to domestic science was the development of food composition tables, which he derived from his own chemical analyses of American food materials as well as from the research he had seen in Germany. Science-minded cooks like Mrs. Lincoln already knew that edibles could be divided into those rich in the "muscle-forming," or "nitrogenous," principle; and those rich in the "heat-producing," or "carbonaceous," principle; but the terms "protein," "carbohydrate," and "fat" were not yet in general use. Atwater made Americans familiar with these terms and also popularized the unit of measurement known as the calorie. In his food composition tables, which began to be published and distributed by the Department of Agriculture in 1895, Atwater listed all the known foods and the amount of protein, carbohydrate, fat, and calories supplied by each. These tables became the building blocks for scientific cookery, and they were most often used in conjunction with Atwater's definition of a standard dietary for Americans. Chemists in England and Germany had already come up with standard dietaries —the amount of nutrients they believed necessary for the body to perform a certain level of work—but Atwater's research into American eating habits, as well as his nationalistic sentiments, convinced him that Americans were different. He recommended less carbohydrate than the German standard, but increased the amount of protein and fat, recognizing and applauding the fact that Americans consumed more milk, meat, eggs, sugar, and butter than Europeans. His standard—125 grams of protein, 125 grams of fat, and 450 grams of carbohydrate for a man "at moderate work"—was not only heartier than that of his European colleagues, it was more than double the amount nutritionists recommend today. "We live more intensely, work harder, need more food, and have more money to buy it," Atwater explained. "The better wages of the American workingman as compared with the European, the larger amount of work he turns off in a day or a year, and his more nutritious food are, I believe, inseparably connected."

Atwater and his students in the domestic-science movement were aware that they still possessed only a partial view of human nutrition, but this awareness did not stop them from putting their ideas before the public with the grand assurance of the enlightened. At heart they were reformers, not research scientists, and they plunged into the practical application of food chemistry without giving any hint of a saving twinge of skepticism. Owing to their self-confidence and sense of publicity, the science of nutrition made a tremendous public splash at the turn of the century. But this was a splash that came too soon for domestic scientists to be able to influence American eating habits as beneficially as they assumed they were doing. Atwater's dietary standard, which reflected his enthusiasm for animal fats and his much lesser regard for fruits and vegetables, was taught and discussed and promoted for over twenty years before the first early news about vitamins began to emerge in 1911. Research on amino acids, similarly, didn't get under way until after the turn of the century and was still rudimentary by World War I. Without a thought to the possible limitations of their knowledge, domestic scientists threw their faith into protein, whether it came in steak or in cornbread. They also persisted in seeing fruits and vegetables as luxury items, both financially and nutritionally, and they admired the way fats and sugars packed a large number of calories into a small amount of food. As late as 1919, in a newspaper article instructing readers how to count calories for a healthy day's food, a cooking teacher with a national reputation wrote a little story about a man who ate snacks from a drugstore one day instead of a proper lunch. When the snacks were viewed scientifically, the teacher explained, they were found to contain more nutrients than a restaurant dinner. Her nutritional analysis of the meal was ingeniously optimistic but typically blind. As the hero explained it, his lunch began with a small package of salted peanuts. "'Let's see—that furnished 500 calories, 100 of them protein calories. To balance the protein I got one ounce of nut milk chocolate for six cents, 181 calories. Then I got a nice big orange for 6 cents. I know it was only 100 calories, but it was half a pound of fruit and neutralized the acid that the chocolate and peanuts produce. And it was so refreshing. Later I had a strawberry college ice for 17 cents with 300 calories. I had really a more nutritious meal than if I had paid $1 for a course dinner and it stayed by me well, too, and only cost 40 cents and no tips.'" This charmed perspective on a balanced diet eventually ran its course, and newer findings in nutrition caught on. But by then domestic scientists—who had become home economists—were no longer identified with dazzling nutritional breakthroughs.

At the height of their reputation, though, teachers of scientific cookery liked nothing better than to take up Atwater's food composition tables and bring them to life in the kitchen. Protein, fat, and carbohydrate became categories to be wielded in the assembling of a rational meal, such as the one devised by the Boston Cooking School for its weekly public lecture-demonstration on December 30, 1896:

Boiled Mutton. *Caper Sauce.*
Mashed Potatoes. *Turkish Pilaf.*
Tomato Fritters. *Cheese Soufflé.*
Cerealine Pudding.

The aim of this sizable winter dinner was to deliver large quantities of protein continuously throughout the meal, beginning with the main course. According to Atwater, mutton was approximately the equivalent of lean beef in terms of protein but was less easily digested on account of its dense, hard fat. The Boston Cooking School recommended long, slow simmering in this case, and added salt halfway through the cooking to enliven an otherwise untouched water broth. The resulting meat, plain but eminently digestible, was assigned a drawn-butter caper sauce in accordance with the usual rules. "Some acid condiment is generally agreeable with meat and fish, owing to the alkaline nature of these substances," Mrs. Lincoln once explained to an *American Kitchen Magazine* subscriber who had written to ask about the correct way to serve sauces. With "more delicate" meats, like lamb and mutton, the acid should be lessened, Mrs. Lincoln went on; hence a "piquant" caper sauce should always adorn mutton, just as mint sauce must appear with lamb. The Turkish pilaf—less adventurous than it sounded, being simply rice browned in butter, steamed in water, and covered with stewed tomatoes—had a secure place here because of the important affinity between mutton and rice. As Atwater had shown, rice offered more protein and carbohydrate than did potatoes, which were largely water, and rice was also more thoroughly digested. On the other hand, nations existing almost entirely on rice were notoriously feeble, so rice needed a powerful protein helpmeet. Sarah Tyson Rorer of the Philadelphia Cooking School was one of the leading defenders of rice, which, as she often pointed out, was digested completely in only one hour. In her magazine *Household News* she personally recommended boiled rice, boiled mutton with caper sauce, and stewed tomatoes as "an exceedingly wise combination." Rice would supply the carbohydrate lacking in the mutton, with the sauce adding a bit of fat, and the acid in the stewed tomatoes hastening the digestion of all. At the Boston Cooking School this combination was buttressed by mashed potatoes, which would linger in the system longer than rice and assure extra heat for the winter. Canned tomatoes were one of the few vegetables available in the winter, and they appeared once more on this menu to create a substantial cold-weather version of a salad—tomato fritters. The tomatoes, cooked with cloves and onion and thickened with cornstarch and an egg, were shaped into croquettes and deep-fried. Since the usual accompaniment to a salad was cheese and crackers, this dinner offered a cheese soufflé with the fritters. The association of cheese with salad was meant to complement quantities of cellulose and water with some protein and fat, so this principle was honored if not exactly realized. The dinner concluded with a dessert that represented a triumph of efficiency and nutritional wisdom. Cerealine was a hot breakfast cereal based on corn, rather like a cornmeal mush; and in the *Boston Cooking-School Cook Book* a recipe for Cerealine pudding was titled "Mock Indian Pudding." Instead of requiring two hours in the oven, as did an authentic Indian pudding, the mock version took only one hour. Nonetheless, the protein in the corn cereal was heavily augmented with milk, carbohydrates were plentiful in the molasses, and the pudding was served with cream to supply the fat, so all the traditional stamina of Indian pudding remained intact.

The manipulation of nutritional components that went on in scientific kitchens was never simply cookery in the minds of its practitioners; it was what an MIT chemist called "external digestion." Cooking was but one stage, and that a late one, in a digestive process that began long before stove or stomach. "The reaping of grain, the capture of animals, the gathering of fruit, the digging of roots or tubers, all are examples of this first great step in digestion," he wrote in a leaflet distributed by domestic scientists at the Chicago World's Fair. Mrs. Lincoln made a similar point during her own speech at the World's Fair: she saw in the very act of digestion "a kind of cooking." As she noted, "Cooking means 'changing by the application of heat,' " a process clearly under way in the workings of the stomach and intestines. Scientific cookery was cookery in the service of digestion, cookery at its most pragmatic, for as Atwater liked to put it (he was translating from the German): "We live upon, not what we eat, but what we digest."

Unlike flavor and appetite, the digestive process was one aspect of eating that was plainly guided by the immutable laws of God, nature, and science, and as such it made an appropriate and dignified centerpiece for any scientific cooking course. No effort in the preparation of food was too extreme if it could be justified with reference to more successful digestion, and digestion timetables were always at hand for use in planning meals. These timetables emerged from a famous series of experiments performed in the 1820s by an American army surgeon named Beaumont who was lucky enough to come across an eighteen-year-old Canadian wounded in a shooting accident. The young man's stomach had been perforated, and the wound left a permanent opening. This inspired Dr. Beaumont to investigate exactly what happened during normal digestion and to induce a variety of artificial conditions as well. By tying a piece of meat to a string and suspending it inside the stomach, Dr. Beaumont was able to mark the rate at which digestive juices did their work; or he could substitute a piece of chicken and compare the rates; or he could feed the young man sour apples and examine the degree of irritation that would build up in the mucous membranes.

The timetables Dr. Beaumont assembled as a result of his observations appeared in cookbooks and women's magazines as well as popular scientific texts, and some of the most influential cooks found them compelling. Sarah Tyson Rorer, who was so fond of rice, in part because of its quick digestion time, carried on a vigorous campaign against the American love of pork, which took five hours to digest. "Life," she used to advise her audiences, "is too short to spend it in digesting pork." Although she occasionally made use of a pork product for variety when putting together her menus, she did so only in the winter months when the body needed extra heat, and then only with elaborate precautions. In January 1894, for instance, she published a menu featuring spare ribs, but carefully scheduled the meal for a Monday—laundry day, when the woman of the family would be doing her hardest work of the week and could best withstand the fat she would encounter at dinnertime. The meal began with a clear soup, which Mrs. Rorer planned specifically for its lack of nutritive properties. The stomach was supposed to simply rest on the soup, gathering strength, as she explained it, "before the heavy work of digesting a spare rib." Applesauce accompanied the spare rib, the acid countering the fat, according to rule, and the side dishes included "cheese ramekins," to give a final spur to the digestive system.

Herbs, spices, condiments, even flavor itself could be understood most satisfactorily by their relation to the digestive process. Ellen Richards analyzed the chemical role of the enjoyment of food in *The Chemistry of Cooking and Cleaning* and concluded that good flavor contributed significantly to assimilation. "Without the appetizing flavor, many a combination of food materials is utterly worthless," she stressed, "for this alone stimulates the desire or appetite, the absence of which may prevent digestion." Overly strenuous flavoring would tax the digestive tract—"like the too frequent and violent application of the whip to a willing steed"—and wear out the glands and membranes. "Just enough to accomplish the purpose is nature's economy," she decided. Atwater was less certain the flavor was crucial, at least in a person of good health, because he knew of laboratory experiments in which tasteless, even repugnant, food was fed to a healthy man, who proceeded to digest it perfectly. In cases of illness, Atwater conceded, the stimulating effect of flavor might well be necessary to activate sluggish organs. Most domestic scientists, who would have had little to do if they had followed Atwater literally on this point, tended to take Mrs. Richards's view. Nevertheless, it would have been highly unusual for them to discuss flavor and appetite in any context other than a physiological one. A physiological context, however, was always on hand if a meal or a recipe seemed to demand a rational explanation. When a reader wrote in to *American Kitchen Magazine* to condemn the large, multicourse dinners that were then fashionable, Mrs. Lincoln—while personally advocating simpler dining—defended the custom by analyzing the digestive function of each course. The meat juices found in soup, along with the dextrin produced by the accompanying roll, would prompt the flow of gastric fluid, hence stimulating the stomach in preparation for its task. Oysters, being quickly absorbed, and delicate white fish that was also easy to assimilate, acted as a sort of warm-up in preparation for the onset of meat and vegetables. The salad, the fruits, the pudding, and the cheese would all make their contribution to "stimulate the nerves of taste," and the chewing required by salted almonds would increase the circulation of blood. In this way a good supply of blood would be furnished to the stomach, and gastric juice would be properly secreted. Mrs. Lincoln advised late afternoon as the safest time for an event on this scale.

These detailed constructions in the physiology of eating, along with the nutritional data constantly appearing in print, came to serve as a kind of map upon which anxious cooks could chart their journeys toward digestion. It was not by any means necessary to attend cooking school in order to practice these maneuvers, for cooking-school methods were described regularly in magazines, lectures, and books aimed at the untutored woman in her kitchen. A woman who had to feed her family on a very modest income, for example, could turn to the *Dietary*

Computer, a pamphlet written by Ellen Richards to serve as a simple guide to planning meals on the basis of food values and cost. Whether or not the economical housekeeper had been trained formally, she could easily refer to Table IV of the *Dietary Computer*, which listed "'Dishes containing meat arranged in order of cost of 100 grams of nitrogenous substance, beginning with the lowest." Among the cheapest meat dishes she would find liver and bacon (under seven cents for one hundred grams of protein, which was close to Atwater's daily minimum for an adult) and roasted beef heart, at seven and a half cents per hundred grams of protein. Choosing perhaps the latter, she would then turn to Table V, which gave one hundred and twenty-nine recipes, and look up No. 11.

NO. 11. ROAST STUFFED HEART WITH VEGETABLES.

Soak the heart in vinegar and water 3 hours, cut off lobes and gristle, stuff with salt, fat pork chopped fine and the same amount of bread crumbs, a little chopped parsley, a little thyme, pepper and salt. Tie in a cloth and let slowly simmer for 2 hours, the larger end up; then take off cloth, flour, and roast until brown with some pieces of pork over it. Make a gravy by thickening with flour.

Every recipe was accompanied by a chart:

	Lbs.	*Oz.*	*Cost.*	*Proteid.*	*Fat.*	*Carb.*	*Cal.*
Heart	3	—	18	231	103	—	1896
Salt							
Fat pork	—	6	3	6	153	—	1447
Crackers	—	4	2	12	12	78	472
Potatoes	2	—	2	16	.8	138	620
Onions	1	—	1	6.8	1.8	40	205
Carrots	1	—	2	4.1	1.3	33	160
Flour	—	1	.15	3.1	.3	21	100
			28.15	279.0	272.2	310	4900

By following the chart exactly, she should be able to supply a family of six with nearly half its necessary protein for the day, paying just over twenty-eight cents. The computer also listed the food values and cost of dishes made with fish, cheese, and eggs, and it included breads, a few vegetables, and desserts. "The recipes are not warranted to succeed the first time trying," Mrs. Richards explained with unusual candor, "but at least, if variations are necessary, the cook will know whether she is increasing or decreasing the food value, which is the chief thing."

Balancing the emphasis on nutritive properties was an equally powerful new interest in the way food looked on the table. Indeed, the dressing up of food, quickly followed by its digestion, provided scientific cooks with a short spectrum of culinary responsibilities that easily bypassed the act of eating. Like the use of spices and condiments, the attractive appearance of a dish was meant to activate the salivary glands, thus assisting the digestive process. Many women attended classes and lectures in scientific cookery especially to see the highly decorated meals that often emerged from cooking-school kitchens, but teachers were careful to justify their work on the basis of gastric stimulation. At the Boston Cooking School special instruction in garnishing and decorating food did not come until after students had mastered the introductory work in "Plain Cooking" and proceeded to "Richer Cooking." Here they encountered in the very first lesson a Boston Cooking School breakfast known as Eggs *à la* Goldenrod, for which they learned to mix hard-boiled egg whites into white sauce, pour the mixture on toast, sprinkle the shredded yolks on top, and garnish with parsley and toast points. "There is probably no meal where attractive table service counts for more than at breakfast," Mrs. Lincoln counseled in *American Kitchen Magazine*. "Appetites are more fickle than after vigorous exercise later in the day." In other lessons cooking students learned to cut vegetables into decorative shapes and float them in consommé, to hide creamed peas inside a potato croquette, to carve tulips out of radishes, to slash the top of a celery stalk so that it would curl backward, and to insert a piece of cold boiled macaroni into the end of a sweetbread-and-mushroom cutlet, possibly to suggest the bone of a chop.

The pinnacle of decorative cooking was the wholly color-coordinated meal, built around the careful selection of flowers, table decorations, and menu items. Cooking-school students were taught to assemble color-coordinated breakfasts, luncheons, and dinners, not only for formal gatherings, but in honor of Valentine's Day (red and white), St. Patrick's Day (green and white), Princeton commencement (orange and black) or Harvard (crimson). Color-coordinated meals enjoyed a surge of popularity among ambitious home cooks as well as cooking students, and ideas were traded back and forth in the pages of the food magazines. Green and white was a frequent combination, since it could be carried out without too much destruction to the food, and Mrs. Lincoln once shared with her readers the description of a green-and-white luncheon created by a subscriber. Grapefruit, lightly covered with white frosting and pistachio nuts, opened the meal; cream of pea soup with whipped cream followed; and the main course was boiled chicken with banana sauce, accompanied by macaroni, creamed spinach, potato balls, and parsley. Green-and-white ices and cakes completed the picture. Other ideas were more adventurous, though not always possible to realize in their entirety—a Bulgarian color scheme put forth one autumn by the *Boston Cooking School Magazine* called for a luncheon decorated heavily with beets, carrots, and egg yolk; and Mrs. Rorer was forced to interrupt an otherwise thoroughly pink meal of strawberries, lobster, and tomatoes with a dish of chicken and peas, since the theme as such lacked sufficient protein. Mrs. Rorer had a special fondness for the all-white meal, which she didn't mind going to some lengths to achieve. Cream soups, cream sauces, boiled poultry, and white fish dominated her dinners, with vanilla ice cream, whipped cream, and angel cake for dessert.

Written up at length in the food magazines, color-coordinated meals were praised for being artistic as well as pragmatic, but what they represented most of all was the achievement of an extraordinary degree of control over the messy, unpredictable business of the kitchen. Good cooking in a turn-of-the-century kitchen was a matter of guesswork even for the experienced. The stove, which burned coal or wood in all but the wealthiest kitchens, could not be adjusted with much certainty: the cook had to gauge the heat by holding her hand in the oven and counting until the heat became unbearable. The quality of flour, butter, eggs, sugar, and other staples could vary bewilderingly from one shopping day to the next, turning a successful dish into a disaster without apparent cause. Printed recipes were always at hand, but they ordinarily conveyed little more than a comfortable hint about the main ingredients. The instructions for Baked Hash that ran in the first issue of *Good Housekeeping* were typically succinct: "Take any kind of cold meat and chop fine with a little cold ham or salt pork; mix in one or two eggs and a little butter and season with salt and pepper; with this, mix bread or rusk crumbs, moisten a very little and bake like a pudding." Most often recipes suggested a "teacupful" of milk, or a "piece of butter the size of an egg"; and frequently they omitted the flour entirely on the assumption that the cook would add enough to make a batter of the "right" consistency.

These problems and conventions, once understood perfectly well by women raised in their mothers' kitchens, had become mysterious barriers to success by the last decades of the nineteenth century. Women wrote constantly to the food magazines wanting to know why dried peaches turned to mush when they were cooked, how to make doughnuts from a recipe that listed no flour, what time of year was best for pickling, what was the difference between corn flour and corn meal, and why the pie crust was a failure. One subscriber was so distraught by the poor texture of her pound cake that she mailed a slice of it to the editor of the *Boston Cooking School Magazine*, begging to know what was wrong. A young housekeeper who was just beginning to be responsible for three meals a day had no assurance that anything she tried to do would turn out right, and even women who had been in the kitchen for years could not predict the results of a day's work with assurance. "Mrs. Tripp has been baking cake this forenoon I have been helping her about it we had splendid luck," wrote a Vermont housemaid in her diary, and in later weeks she recorded their success with pineapple preserves and squash pies, always attributing it to "splendid luck."

Nothing infuriated the most scientific cooks so much as the thought of luck ruling the kitchen. Helen Campbell, an enthusiastic social reformer in the domestic-science movement, complained to an audience at the University of Wisconsin that "even the intelligent housekeeper still talks about 'luck with her sponge cake.' *Luck!* There is no such word in science, and to make sponge cake is a scientific process!" Cooking teachers were vigorous in their efforts to discredit any notion of the erratic or spontaneous in the kitchen, and to assure every student that she ruled absolutely. " 'The only things I consider beyond my control in cooking are the wind and weather,' " asserted one teacher, " 'which affect the drafts of the range.' " If the housekeeper could be made to think of herself as a scientist, calmly at work over the beakers and burners in her laboratory, then every meal would emerge as she planned, pristine and invariable. "There is no reason why the cook should not be as sure of her results as is a chemist," argued another teacher. "When the druggist has a prescription to fill he does not mix his ingredients in a haphazard manner, trusting to luck that it will come out all right; but everything is carefully weighed and measured and put together in just the right way, and then he knows exactly what the result will be." The smooth, intelligible flow of tasks that made up a chemist's workday as these teachers imagined it became the model for scientific cookery. Cooking-school rules and procedures were designed to ensure as rigidly as possible the right result—a meal perfect in all its proportions—not only under laboratory conditions, but in every American home. Most women wouldn't have identified themselves as chemists, perhaps, but many responded gladly to the promise of order and rationality that came with scientific cookery.

The starting point in scientific cookery was most often a specific menu, rather than a specific food. Traditionally a European or American housekeeper would have fed her family according to the season and the local economy, bringing into the kitchen perhaps a loin of beef, from which she would extract, during the week, an array of different meals—steaks, stews, chopped meat, soups, and broth. A few of the cooking authorities at the turn of the century still coached their readers and students in this skill, but it was becoming less necessary except on farms and in isolated villages. Women who lived in cities and suburbs and could shop easily were learning a different, more refined approach: to assemble nutritionally based eating plans and then to buy only what was needed for each dish. The practicality of European housekeepers, who continued to organize their meals from the point of view of the food at hand, was much praised by domestic scientists. But what they understood best from their impressions of French and German cookery came to little more than the importance of using up leftovers, a theme they cherished. Too intimate a contact with food, too many spontaneous ways in the kitchen, simply raised their suspicions. And while they were heavily dependent upon recipes, they showed little interest in collecting quantities of them on the basis of gustatory novelty alone. Scientific cooks preferred to stand back and assess an entire meal, or better still an entire day or week of nutritional intake. Menu making, when it was undertaken in a properly analytical frame of mind, was the educated woman's approach to the kitchen. Whether or not a woman had servants who could take over the manual labor of cookery, she could always keep hold of her dignity and her intellect if she started with a written rationale. When the Help-One-Another Club, an advice column that ran regularly in *The Woman's Home Companion*, announced an essay contest on the topic "What I Have for Breakfast, and Why," readers from all over the country mailed in their breakfast menus, with essays that ardently demonstrated their commitment to scientific meal planning. The first prize went to a

Jackson, Mississippi, woman who submitted seven breakfasts, all emphasizing mastication ("the strength and formation of the teeth depend in a great measure on the chewing of the food") and ease of digestion. An Ohio reader who sent in two menus organized specifically against constipation ("the bane of humanity") won a dollar; her breakfasts featured raw fruit, stewed corn, baked potatoes, and hot water. Another woman, writing from upstate New York, testified that "tumbled hair, soiled wrappers and dragging shoestrings" were never seen at her breakfast table. "Cheerful faces, clean attire, nourishing but light breakfasts, carefully prepared and served, go a long way toward morals!" she advised. Several menus displayed dishes like creamed potatoes, minced beef, or hash, to demonstrate the economical use of leftovers; and two readers made a point of criticizing fresh, hot breads and griddle cakes ("an abomination," "a tax on the digestion"), since virtually all domestic-science authorities agreed that such preparations could never be digested adequately. A Minnesota reader did admit that her family ate doughnuts for breakfast ("We do not claim that they are strictly hygienic") but added by way of apology that she had been raised in New England, where pies and doughnuts were an old-fashioned custom in the morning. Some writers found it harder than others to come up with a scientific rationale for their breakfasts. The most desperate was probably the Vermont woman who tried to justify poached eggs on toast with the explanation "Eggs in any form are agreeable to every one in general," and praised melons for their "humidity."

Menus that spelled out the complete food for a family, covering up to a month at a time, were a consistently popular feature in the cookery and women's magazines. The editors of *New England Kitchen Magazine* resisted the trend for several years after beginning publication, feeling that menus, like too many fancy recipes, might be overstimulating. Holding themselves aloof from those magazines and newspapers that regularly filled their pages with new recipes, Mrs. Lincoln and Anna Barrows noted that their own serious-minded readers seemed happy enough "to learn principles rather than new dishes." Eventually, however, they gave in to what must have been mounting demand and began printing a week's worth of suggested menus in each issue—but "simple, practical every day dishes," Mrs. Lincoln emphasized, "those that people really have." Mrs. Lincoln's own tastes, hearty but somewhat toneless, predominated in these menus, and a succession of bananas, baked beans, stewed fruit, and numerous potatoes marched with stolid predictability through the magazine's bills of fare. Taking pains to avoid French-sounding dishes, extravagance in any form, and the slightest hint of impertinence, she set up her eating plans on the basis of washday (Monday), ironing day (Tuesday), maid's day off (Thursday), and day of relative rest (Sunday). A suitably quick but substantial lunch for women at home doing the laundry on a Monday in April, for example, would be potato salad, bread, and oranges, especially if enough potatoes were boiled at midday to ensure leftovers for dinner, and invariably they were. Potato salad, in these pages, regularly signaled mashed potatoes for dinner. On Tuesday, when she felt most people wanted only those dishes that did not "scent the clean clothes with the odor of onions or frying," she came up with a triumphantly scent-free meal of baked-bean soup, dry toast, and stewed raisins. Mrs. Lincoln also tried to balance heavy foods with light, and large noon meals with simple, easily digested suppers. If a massive noon dinner seemed in order—baked beans, baked potatoes, and baked Indian pudding were all assembled for one weighty November luncheon—the day would be completed with a supper as light as she could possibly make it, in this case popcorn and milk.

Printed menus in the magazine were usually accompanied by a selection of recipes and sometimes by detailed plans of action, meant to guide the housekeeper from meal to meal. These work plans emphasized above all the precise dispersal of leftovers, an accomplishment that became a crucial link from one meal to the next.

"The liver terrapin is made, of course, from that left over from larded liver, and is one of the daintiest of luncheon dishes," Mrs. Rorer explained to the readers of *Household News*, discussing the first Tuesday and Wednesday in July. (*Household News* had the economical habit of printing menus only for the first two weeks of each month, on the assumption that readers could simply repeat the entire process to complete the month.)

> Now, on Friday you have sauce tartar; yolk of one egg will be quite sufficient, and for dinner mayonnaise will take two, and sauce hollandaise two more, so you will have five whites for your sponge gems on Saturday. . . . You will probably have more chopped meat than you want for meat cakes, especially if you add also the bits of lean meat from bones and sirloin steaks. This can be used for smothered beef Sunday morning. The bones must be placed at once in the soup kettle, covered with cold water, and cooked slowly for four hours to make clear soup for Sunday dinner, and macaroni soup for Monday.

Whether or not too many women followed with exactitude the menus and schedules that cooking authorities prepared for them, an abundance of written information became lodged in the American kitchen, and housekeepers grew accustomed to a kind of buffer zone of print between themselves and the raw food. Rather than learning to consult their instincts, their sense of taste, or their imaginations, fledgling cooks were taught to depend on rules, which existed on a lofty plane far above the pleasures of appetite. Even the homely, practical advice of a mother or grandmother was too primitive to be taken seriously any longer. "Housekeeping handed down by tradition becomes narrow and empirical," observed Anna Barrows. ". . . Heretofore there has been no defined standard of good housekeeping; 'my way is the right way' has been the unspoken rule with this as with religious matters." To domestic scientists, the inchoate nature of traditional cookery was a sorry reminder of humankind's barbaric past. They liked to think of "man" as the "cooking animal" and of cookery as the great civilizing force in human history. In this view, raw food was a foreign, slightly menacing substance that had to be brought under strict control before it could meet the scientifically ascertained needs of the modern American family. "The savage tears his food, and often eats it raw," commented an editorial in the *Boston Cooking School Magazine*. "As he emerges from barbarism more refined ways are practiced."

One of the major civilizing influences in the American kitchen was widely recognized to be white sauce. In most cooking schools the making of white sauce out of flour, butter, and milk, especially to pour over boiled potatoes, comprised an early lesson, in part because both potatoes and sauce illustrated with obvious drama the action of heat upon starch, and in part because white sauce was as basic to cooking-school cookery as the stove itself. There was virtually no cooked food that at one time or another was not hidden, purified, enriched, or ennobled with white sauce—among scientific cooks it became the most popular solution to the discomfiting problem of undressed food. According to Mrs. Lincoln, parsnips, turnips, cabbage, and celery should all be served in white sauce, and even the humble carrot—"not a favorite vegetable for the table"—could be rendered acceptable by being served the same way. Unappetizing winter beets, advised *Harper's Bazaar*, should be boiled all day, then reheated the next day and offered with white sauce. Anna Barrows simply made a general recommendation that all vegetables, "when they were covered up with this white sauce," would be eaten gladly by people who otherwise disliked them. At the Boston Cooking School, women attending a lecture-demonstration in February 1897 were shown how to prepare the new "Frankfort sausages": they were to be boiled and served with white sauce. A turkey garnished with white sauce was among the "Seasonable Dishes for January" described in *American Kitchen Magazine*, and Mrs. Lincoln liked to drench pieces of steamed halibut in white sauce, decorating them with thick slices of hard-boiled egg. Sarah

Tyson Rorer once advised sinking a boiled chicken into a bed of popcorn and smothering the whole thing in white sauce. Her successor as the editor of *Table Talk*, a cooking teacher named Cornelia C. Bedford, was so captivated by white sauce that in the menus she scheduled for one memorable day—August 4, 1899—she included it at every meal: for breakfast, on panned tomatoes; for lunch, on clams sautés; and for dinner, on egg cutlets. Queried by a subscriber about what to do when unexpected company arrived, Mrs. Lincoln answered by recounting one of her own experiences, in which she received three sudden guests with only a few scraps of ham, two oranges, and two bananas in the house. White sauce was the chief agent in transforming these remnants into "an ample and satisfactory luncheon." And in 1891 a Mormon woman, traveling to a new home in Nevada with her husband and five children, stopped along the way to stay overnight with another of her husband's wives. "Among other things she served alfalfa greens dressed with white sauce," recalled the pioneer in her memoirs. "It was quite a tasty dish."

The standard recipe—or as some teachers preferred to think of it, the "formula"—called for two tablespoons of butter, two tablespoons of flour, and a cup of milk. Essentially this white sauce was a béchamel without benefit of flavoring, but American scientific cooks stopped short of putting their white sauce to work in the French manner. The important function of an American white sauce was not to enhance but to blanket. The addition of different flavors and textures to the basic formula was an impressive next step largely on account of its marvelous efficiency, which cooking teachers loved to describe. Lecturing to a Minnesota audience, Juliet Corson of the New York Cooking School first made a pint of white sauce and then went on to detail the variations that were possible. With sugar, it became "a nice pudding sauce." A tablespoon of chopped parsley would turn it into parsley sauce. A few capers would create caper sauce, and a teaspoonful of anchovies transformed it into anchovy sauce. Miss

Corson was right, to an extent, but her view of sauce making penetrated no deeper than the surface of the dish. To assemble a sauce from the food outward, to link it with the rest of the dish because certain elements of both were compatible or perhaps surprising, would have demanded the kind of gustatory intensity that scientific cooks were determined to leave behind them. In a series of cooking lessons printed in the *Boston Cooking School Magazine*, sauce making was introduced as a kind of kitchen tool used occasionally to make food more functional. "Often richness or moisture, one or both, would improve an article of food, and, sometimes, we wish to add to the bulk of certain articles to make them 'go farther,'" wrote the editor. "In either case we may have recourse to sauces." In this spirit, white sauce became a substitute for imaginative composition, not a factor in it. When Miss Corson came to the subject of meat, therefore, she advised her Minnesota audience to boil pieces of veal, then make a white sauce using the broth, and finally add an egg yolk and some chopped parsley to the mixture. The result would be, she assured them, "a dish called in French cookery books *blanquette*. . . ." Here was a *blanquette de veau* that shot straight to its point, with no extraneous gestures in the way of cream, onions, mushrooms, or seasonings. Similarly, when Sarah Tyson Rorer dipped pieces of cooked chicken into her white sauce, she unhesitatingly called the dish a "*chaud-froid*" —briskly dispensing with the glaze and seasonings that characterized the traditional version.

This fondness for whitening their food before eating it became a habit that cooks extended to soups, salads, and desserts. Creamy sauces and garnishes were prescribed consistently in the menus they wrote up, so that soups arrived with whipped cream atop each bowl, tossed salads were smeared with boiled dressings or with mayonnaise mixed with whipped cream, and ice creams and Bavarian creams turned up for dessert covered with more cream. White ways to extend and reheat leftovers, as with creamed fish and creamed potatoes, were already traditional in American kitchens; in the scientific kitchen they multiplied profusely. "The secret of a successful *réchauffé* is its complete disguise," wrote a California woman to the Help-One-Another Club. "It should be combined with other ingredients, seasoned, and served so that its identity is completely lost." White sauce performed this task often. Many dinners emerging from the scientific kitchen were entirely white, not just on the special occasions that called for an all-white meal, but in the course of an ordinary week. Boiled cod, mashed potatoes, rice, and macaroni pudding were the components of a meal featured in the first issue of the *Ladies' Home Journal.* Two months later the magazine suggested serving boiled chicken with macaroni, whipped potato, creamed parsnips, and—to brighten things up slightly—"Jonquil Blanc-mange." The kitchen itself was becoming whiter by the turn of the century. Announcing as it did a pure and germ-free environment, whiteness became the prevailing aesthetic in kitchens and bathrooms, where walls and fixtures could be painted to display the outward sign of inner sanitation.

Even the cook was supposed to be able to emerge from the kitchen looking as unsullied as possible, as if she had prepared the dinner without touching it. During the 1894 World's Food Fair, an exposition for manufacturers and retailers in the food industry, *New England Kitchen Magazine* praised at length the "daintiness and deftness" of the cooking-school graduates who were in charge of many of the exhibits and did the public cookery demonstrations. "There should be less objection on the part of many to going into the kitchen after seeing these young women make bread, fry fishballs, arrange a salad or mix a cake, without injury to a fresh and becoming dress," the magazine commented. "Too many women think an ugly or shabby attire is a necessity in the kitchen. The brigade of cooks and attendants in dainty gowns, white aprons and caps, doing their work of mixing, cooking and serving, without making a 'mess' of themselves or their surroundings, teach a lesson that many, surely, note and follow."

The enveloping mask of smoothness and purity that each portion of white sauce brought to bear on the food beneath represented a kind of cookery that had been lifted beyond drudgery to a plane of harmony and order. Cooking teachers taught their pupils techniques that would help them tame food, rather than bring it to life, and the resulting dishes tended to be laden with the evidence of this domestication. The problem of vegetables and salad ingredients was particularly challenging, since the very existence of these foods seemed to defy rational analysis. Until the identification of vitamins, only those vegetables offering a useful amount of protein, carbohydrate, or fat—namely peas, beans, lentils, and potatoes—had a dietary function that could be considered legitimate. Plainly, green and yellow vegetables added a necessary bulk to the diet, but beyond that it was difficult to define their function, even though most cooking authorities sensed their value. "Vegetables are rich in saline substances which counteract the evil effect of too much animal food," was Mrs. Lincoln's guess. "Some are rich in organic acids, and many abound in indigestible ligneous tissues which are useful in certain conditions." Other cooks also attributed the elusive function of vegetables to "salts"—by which they usually meant minerals —or "mild acids" that helped in the digestion of protein. "Last, but not least, they are pleasing to the eye . . ." explained one atypical writer, "since with their gayer colors they are apt to relieve the sober hues of the meats."

A thorough scrubbing followed by an equally thorough boiling was the usual prescription for vegetables, which had to be cooked long past the point of resistance in order to be deemed digestible. According to the syllabus for one cooking course, it was primitive "man's" first encounter with a vegetable that prompted his rise from savagery. Fruits and nuts he could consume raw, but the moment he saw a vegetable he understood that it had to be boiled, and at that moment he took his first step toward civilization. Most authorities recommended one to three hours' boiling for string beans, forty-five minutes for asparagus, twenty minutes for cucumbers, half an hour for celery, and up to twelve hours for beets. Crispness, crunchiness, even the springy texture of freshness itself, were sensations in which these cooks apparently had no wish to indulge. With a heavy blanket of white sauce they completed their refurbishing of cooked vegetables.

Salad greens, which did have to be served raw and crisp, demanded more complicated measures. The object of scientific salad making was to subdue the raw greens until they bore as little resemblance as possible to their natural state. If a plain green salad was called for, the experts tried to avoid simply letting a disorganized pile of leaves drop messily onto the plate. One cook recommended cutting the lettuce leaves into "ribbons of uniform width" for a more orderly arrangement, and the most popular version of a spinach salad required the spinach to be boiled, drained, chopped, molded into little cups, unmolded, and decorated with a neat slice of hard-boiled egg. The same precision was appropriate even for a tossed lettuce salad, as Mrs. Lincoln once explained to a Denver audience. By following her directions, a hostess would be able to take control of any lettuce salad in full view of company.

> Arrange the lettuce in a salad bowl, the outer leaves on the edge and so on, the small ones all in the middle and the edges up so that it will have the effect of a head of lettuce fully open [Mrs. Lincoln instructed]. Put at the left of the hostess a small, shallow, fancy bowl in which to mix the dressing. . . . At her right place the oil, vinegar, salt, pepper and mustard. . . . Pour it over the lettuce, letting it touch every leaf, if possible. Then with the salad spoon and fork, or two forks, if you have no salad set, turn the leaves over and over until all are saturated with the dressing.
>
> After a little practice one may do this so deftly that the leaves will be left in nearly the same shape as at first.

This arduous approach to salad making became an identifying feature of cooking-school cookery and the signature of a refined household. "Dainty" and "refreshing" were the adjectives most often used to describe salads, and they were perceived as the appropriate food for people who needed something other than blunt, substantial calories from their meals. Students, professionals, office employees, and others in the expanding white-collar class known as "brain-workers" were supposed to prefer light, easily assimilated foods that would leave their minds clear and active. The presence of salad on a menu became an effective way to distinguish the meal as one meant for the wealthy, or at least the ambitious middle class, which could afford relatively expensive ingredients wrought into a cajoling design. The author of *Progressive Housekeeping* advised her readers somewhat daringly that they could avoid the trouble of planning two different meals if they served the same midday dinner to both servants and family members. But she was careful to note, in describing a few menus that would be suitable, that when salad was included she meant it solely for "upstairs" and on those occasions the "downstairs" table should have pickles instead. Salads were so strongly identified with the upper ranks of society that even in families employing a cook, the lady of the house was expected to make the salads herself. "Surely no lady who has a hand and knows how to use it deftly and gracefully would be willing to relinquish this most fascinating part of the dinner service . . ." remarked Mrs. Lincoln; and another authority stressed, "I never allow a servant even to touch the leaves of the salad I have served at table, for to have the salad to perfection the touch must be light, the fingers to trim and arrange must be nimble."

American salads traditionally had been a matter of fresh greens, chicken, or lobster, but during the decades at the turn of the century, when the urban and suburban middle class was beginning to define itself, salads proliferated magnificently in number and variety until they incorporated nearly every kind of food except bread and pastry, which were occasionally used to hold them. Any preparation that could be served on a lettuce leaf eventually was, and dishes that once would have been treated as savories or desserts took on new importance and dignity as salads. Squares of frozen cream cheese were a salad; hard-boiled egg yolks mashed with mayonnaise, formed into balls and rolled in cottage cheese, were a Golf Salad; fruits that had been frozen into a mold lined with mayonnaise and whipped cream were a Salad Mousse or a Frozen Fruit Salad; a pear half with slivers of almond piercing it was a Porcupine Salad, and any combination of apples, nuts, celery, pineapple, and mayonnaise made a loose version of the enormously popular Waldorf Salad, introduced soon after the hotel opened in 1893.

Salads that were nothing but a heap of raw ingredients in disarray plainly lacked cultivation, and the cooking experts developed a number of ingenious ways to wrap them up. The lettuce "cup" became a prominent device in scientific salad making, for it could hold an individual serving of salad without the problem of loose, sprawling leaves. *Home Science Cook Book* recommended that its readers ignore entirely the messier varieties of lettuce and choose only "close, firm, solid heads" with their "crisp, cup-shaped inner leaves." Other popular ways to keep the salad course attractively within bounds included the apple-celery-and-mayonnaise salad packed into a tomato; a banana-and-nut salad tucked inside a banana skin; a spoonful of marinated peas held in a hollowed-out boiled turnip; and a fruit salad walled in by four crackers standing on edge, the whole tied about with a ribbon. A ring cut from a red pepper could be used to confine spears of asparagus, and a string-bean salad could be hidden within a "crown" made of hard-boiled eggs that had been cut in quarters lengthwise. The pieces of egg had to be trimmed so that each would stand level, and they were stuck to the plate with gelatin. Mrs. Lincoln once commented favorably upon a celery salad that was wholly subjugated by being served in a block of ice ("very artistic"), but she made no attempt to describe how it was supposed to be freed and eaten.

The tidiest and most thorough way to package a salad was to mold it in gelatin. American cooks were already accustomed to making fruit and wine jellies, or serving a decorative main dish such as boned turkey in aspic, and for these preparations they used either commercial gelatin or a homemade calf's-foot jelly. The former, while more convenient, was available only shredded or in sheets, and needed to soak half an hour or longer before it was ready to use. In 1893 Sarah Tyson Rorer wrote to the Knox company suggesting that they produce their gelatin in granulated form, which would be easier to measure and would dissolve more quickly. A year later Knox began advertising a "Sparkling Granulated Gelatine," and offering to send upon request a copy of the recipe booklet "Dainty Desserts for Dainty People." Other manufacturers quickly imitated the innovation, and within the decade flavored granulated gelatins had been introduced as well. At first the new product was used much as the old shredded gelatins had been—to make puddings, mousses, charlottes, and jellies, as well as the occasional main dish, or tomato aspic—but the possibilities for salad making soon became evident. "This is dainty for company," suggested a contributor to *New England Kitchen Magazine*, and gave directions for a cheese salad that she made by adding granulated gelatin to a boiled dressing, then folding in whipped cream and grated cheese, and molding the mixture in egg cups for individual servings. Mayonnaise, which scientific cooks had tended to spread as a cloak over the surface of a salad, now could be easily stiffened with gelatin and used to harden a chicken salad that had been shaped to look like a chop, with a bit of almond representing the bone. "Could you give directions for a jelly where pieces of oranges, bananas, white grapes, are used and are seen in the jelly?" wrote a Connecticut subscriber to Mrs. Lincoln in 1896. Mrs. Lincoln explained how to mold the fruits in layers of orange gelatin; a few years later the same fruit jelly appeared in the magazine as a salad. Shortly after the turn of the century there emerged a gelatin salad that crowned all these achievements, for it captured, confined, and molded raw vegetables themselves. This was the Perfection Salad, a mixture of cabbage, celery, and red peppers, all chopped fine and bound by a plain aspic. During the next decades there was only one notable change in the recipe—the plain aspic became tomato—while the other straightforward ingredients hardly altered. Unlike the Waldorf Salad, which in the course of becoming an institution was elaborated in any number of extraordinary ways, the Perfection Salad firmly maintained its identity, the very image of a salad at last in control of itself.

Despite the often hefty ingredients that were assembled in its name, the salad course never lost its original image as a fragile, leafy interlude that was something of a nutritional frill. As a kind of non-food, the salad course had a non-nutritive function: it enhanced the femininity of the whole meal and made the scientific cook herself more socially palatable. Decorative, seemingly ephemeral, salads were perceived as ladies' food, reflecting the image of frailty attached to the women who made them. Ever since the opening of the Boston Cooking School, when the committee had discussed for hours the problem of how to dispose of the food that would be cooked in class, domestic scientists had taken for granted that eating food was a great deal less feminine than preparing it. The general management of food did appear to them to be an intrinsically female preoccupation, but even the most progressive of the scientific cooks would have hesitated to assign so vehement a trait as physical appetite to a lady. The proper number of calories was just as important for a woman to achieve as it was for a man, but menus planned for women always emphasized sweet, ethereal foods, some of them almost imperceptible as nourishment. "Edible Flowers," "A Mermaid's Dinner," and "A Butterfly Luncheon" were among the most-talked-about table displays created by a local cooking teacher for the 1894 Food Fair in Boston; and ornamental salads and desserts were abundant in the menus for ladies' luncheons that ran constantly in the food magazines. These luncheons rarely came closer to red meat than an occasional lamb chop. A Boston lecture-demonstration entitled "Foods That Tickle the Feminine Palate" began with three entrees incorporating eggs and fish, and then devoted itself to fudge, caramels, fruit salad with marshmallows, and an elaborate ice cream coupe. The assumption that women were averse to meat—or ought to be—was widespread, and indeed helped give rise to a virtual epidemic of iron-deficiency anemia among adolescent girls, which lasted until after the turn of the century. Affecting the languor and the wandering appetite they associated with femininity, girls of all social classes would refuse meat in favor of pastries and bread. Their disease was known as chlorosis—the "green sickness"—and although it was not well understood medically at the time, it was at least considered an illness, despite the fact that the pallor of the girls suffering from it was often called beautiful. No such mixed reaction was in order when the same eating habits were observed in boys, however. Margaret Sidney, the author of *Five Little Peppers*, wrote a prize-winning essay for *Good Housekeeping* entitled "How to Eat, Drink, and Sleep as a Christian Should," in which she described the anguish of a hypothetical family whose son showed the unmistakable symptoms of femininity in his food preferences. Young Tom, she wrote,

> looks and acts just like a girl. It is a more difficult task for the little mother to feed him, and father often looks up from his own dinner or thinks it over during his hard day's work at the office, wondering if "mother" is on the right track. Both parents know that Tom should be helped up to a sturdy boyhood; not having all his girlish fancies indulged. How can they make him love the rare, juicy tender roast beef, and the hot baked potato that he now turns from, holding in his hunger until the pudding gets on the table?

By contrast with ladies' luncheons, the dinners planned for men were mighty, sometimes blatant, symbols of maleness. Commonly recommended for a bachelor supper or a men's-club dinner were saddle of mutton, woodcock, strong cheese, brown bread, and hard crackers. When the Boston Cooking School presented a lecture called "What Husbands Like to Eat," the overwhelming choices were fried rabbit, baked stuffed eggplant, potatoes baked in a casserole, spiced cheese, and a pâté with chili peppers. A lettuce salad did appear on this menu, but lest the greens seem too fragile for such a masculine occasion, they were weighed down with an oil-and-vinegar dressing to which a scoop of Colonel Skinner's Chutney had been added. The lettuce course was then anchored beyond all doubt by an entire baked ham—"Have this passed with the salad," were the lecturer's instructions.

The mission of a scientific cook was to nourish all the members of the family adequately and appropriately, but by far the most popular dishes in cooking-school classes and public demonstrations were the ones that emphasized a highly recognizable femininity and put up a firm aesthetic barrier around the food. "It is too artistic to eat!" was the compliment uttered by an audience member at one of Mrs. Lincoln's salad demonstrations, after she passed around a potato salad laden with shredded egg white, shredded yolk, rows of parsley, borders of "crisp, inner lettuce leaves," and a small heap of shredded beets. Food that could be appreciated most fully without being eaten was a special achievement in scientific cookery, which had its own aesthetic principles. Croquettes, timbales, creamed foods served in pastry shells or ramekins, molded desserts—anything that could be encapsulated, or made smaller and prettier than life, became a recurring favorite. When Brussels sprouts came on the market, they were greeted with delight as miniature cabbages. At a Boston Cooking School dinner-menu demonstration held in March 1898, every dish except the introductory bowl of soup showed the effort to disguise food, reduce its volatility, keep it within visible borders: the fish was molded and served with cream sauce; the chicken was baked in a casserole; stuffed pimentos were placed on toast and covered with white sauce; a Neufchâtel Salad was made of diced cheese on lettuce; and the dessert was a frozen pudding.

Undoubtedly the most familiar sign of aesthetically correct cookery was the chafing dish, which soared into popularity in the 1890s and quickly established a method of food preparation so tidy and refined that it could happen right at the dinner table. If the ingredients were chopped and measured beforehand and arranged on the table at the hostess's place, she could mix a simple sauce in the chafing dish, perhaps add some eggs or leftover pieces of meat, heat them a few moments, and serve the meal—all without dirtying her hands, since it was possible to almost completely avoid touching the food. Like the elaborately tossed salad described by Mrs. Lincoln, which was supposed to look in the end as though it had never been tossed at all, a chafing-dish meal could be prepared by a woman who hardly seemed to be cooking, so distant was she from the intimation of raw food. Hence the use of the chafing dish did not by any means identify the cook as a servant or a drudge. "Kate Douglas Wiggin and Mary E. Wilkins are said to be enthusiasts over chafing dish cookery," noted *American Kitchen Magazine*, naming two of the most beloved writers of the day, "and many other literary women are of the same mind." Chafing-dish cookery was so far above ordinary kitchen duties that even men might be supposed to take an interest in it, and menus for bachelor suppers regularly suggested that the host preside over a chafing dish. "We have looked upon the chafing dish as a missionary in disguise," *American Kitchen Magazine* editorialized, "which would induce many young women to a more thorough study of combinations of foods." All the famous cooking teachers lectured frequently on the chafing dish and produced cookbooks devoted to it, and at the Boston Cooking

School, students sometimes wore a little pin with a picture of a chafing dish on it. It was the school's official brooch.

The distinction between an educated cook and a drudge was crucial to establish, and scientific cookery at its most refined was able to both lift and clarify the status of the woman in charge of the kitchen. "This lesson shows that it takes ladies and artists to do work of this kind," remarked an appreciative member of the audience as Mrs. Lincoln demonstrated her salads. Cooking-school methods were attractive for what they offered the cook, as much as for what they did to the food; and if cooking schools did not always create professionals, they certainly never failed to graduate ladies. The importance of this identity for the woman in the kitchen was acknowledged by *Good Housekeeping* right at the outset of its long presence in American homes. In an immensely popular serial that started shortly after the magazine began publication in 1885, an ambitious young bride named Molly Bishop sets up housekeeping determined that she will never look messy or haggard when her husband comes home, for he is afraid that the hard work is going to exhaust her and give her the rough red hands of a servant. Molly does manage to change her dress and arrive fresh and sweet at the dinner table each night, but back in the kitchen there is a hired girl who is just her opposite—Marta, the "stupid-looking" German servant, who shuffles around in thick-soled slippers. An immigrant who speaks no English, Marta cannot stone an olive without tearing it and would have instinctively tumbled all the biscuits into a dish in disarray had not Molly taken pains to show her how to arrange them nicely. Aware that Marta, newly arrived in America, "could not have been accustomed to doing things daintily," Molly gives the girl patient instruction, but the differences between the two cooks in the Bishop kitchen remain vivid. Molly takes care to retain her soft white hands; she also notices that she is more frail than Marta, and tires more quickly than the sturdy German. Furthermore, Molly applies her cooking-school education to every aspect of cookery from precise measuring to pretty serving, while Marta, heavy and clumsy, knows only the most bumbling country ways of doing things and has never even seen a written recipe.

Molly's educated and well-bred ways in the kitchen not only distinguish her effectively from the woman working alongside her but they pay off splendidly. Her husband's rich parents, who had rejected him when he married "pretty, penniless Molly" instead of the wealthy Miss Vanderpool, are so impressed by Molly's simple but ladylike cookery that they restore the young couple to favor. This fairy-tale ending, while gratifying, could not have come as much of a surprise to the readers of *Good Housekeeping*, who would have been able to see easily through Molly's humble surroundings to the lady of fortune waiting to be released. The culinary clues are frequent—they begin to appear with the very first lunch prepared by Molly for her husband, which features a chicken salad carefully masked by mayonnaise—and one of the broadest hints is dropped in the chapter on cabbage. Heavy and strong-smelling, boiled cabbage was not a food associated with the best households, and when Molly expresses a desire for it, her husband is shocked ("You vulgar little person!") But at dinnertime there is no odor of boiled cabbage in the house, and when her husband sits down he finds a dish of mild, creamy cabbage in front of him, dressed in a white sauce and as easily digested as a sprig of parsley. The secret of refined cabbage—"*rapid boiling, plenty of water, plenty of room, and the cover off*"—is no secret to Molly. She may have been brought up in a cottage, but as she declares to her husband early in the serial: " 'I assure you, I haven't been to cooking schools for nothing.' "

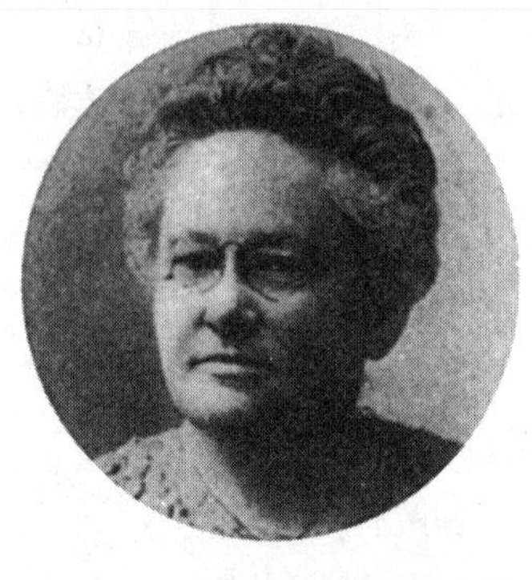

Five
The Mother of Level Measurements

Most of the private cooking schools that attracted attention at the turn of the century had faded from notice by the time the country was engaged in World War I. To the extent that scientific cookery was a fad it ended at that time, but as a new and more challenging way for women to think about life in the kitchen, it reigned for another half century. A good many social and commercial trends contributed to the long flourishing of the scientific kitchen, but the chief culinary source for its vigor was Fannie Merritt Farmer, the best-known cooking teacher of her era and the only one whose name is still famous today. Fannie Farmer was not without competitors, but throughout her career she was recognized as a remarkable leader in a crowded field. Unlike many of her colleagues she never claimed to be an advanced scientist, a philosopher, or a moral guide; instead, she liked to think of herself as a businesswoman. Her product was scientific cookery and she had complete faith in it; what she was able to do better than anybody else, finally, was to make it accessible, appealing, and even necessary to middle-class housekeepers.

In the winter of 1905 *The Woman's Home Companion*

invited each of six notable cooks to submit a column entitled "My Twelve Favorite Recipes." Cookbook authors Marion Harland and her daughter Christine Terhune Herrick, both of them already regular contributors to the *Companion*, were selected; Mrs. Lincoln, as the editor of *New England Kitchen Magazine*, and Janet McKenzie Hill, who edited the *Boston Cooking School Magazine*, were both invited; Elizabeth O. Hiller of the Chicago Domestic Science Cooking School was included; and the sixth was Fannie Farmer, at that time principal of Miss Farmer's School of Cookery. After all six of the columns had run, the editors announced that from then on Miss Farmer would write regularly and exclusively for the *Companion*—"something which every progressive housekeeper has been looking forward to. . . ." With her twelve favorite recipes Miss Farmer had managed to outstrip several of the most important authorities of the day, in particular distancing herself from Mrs. Lincoln, whose twelve favorites were determined by a stated desire for "hygienic living." In her column Mrs. Lincoln explained that she always avoided "rich foods" and dishes "overpowered by sauces and condiments." Lamb chops standing around a mound of mashed potatoes, molded spinach with its garnish of egg, a Waldorf Salad stuffed into a green pepper, and "poor man's" rice pudding were among her characteristically mild suggestions. Fannie Farmer, on the other hand, added oysters and canned tomatoes to dress up a classic French bouillon; she made fish fillets and timbales and drenched them in rich sauces; she put a paper frill on her cheese croquettes; and she created two major salads. Harvard Salad was made with chopped chicken in a whipped-cream dressing, packed into a basket that had been carved from a lemon, and decorated with parsley and—for the school's "crimson"—infinitesimal parings of radish skin. For Brazilian Salad she combined Brazil nuts with grapes, pineapple, celery, and mayonnaise, stationing each serving in its own little pen made of four saltines. Miss Farmer's selection was rounded out powerfully with sweets: chocolate pudding, chocolate sauce, caramel bisque ice cream, and a birthday cake.

Whether or not these recipes really were her personal favorites—it seems likely they were—they ranked high indeed with her followers.

Fannie Farmer was born in Boston in 1857 and grew up in the nearby town of Medford. Her mother had been born in Boston, too, and always considered that city a birthplace of special distinction. Mary Watson Merritt Farmer was known as a "notable housewife," at least according to one of Fannie's eulogies. A niece in the family remembered Mrs. Farmer looking dubiously at her daughter's culinary experiments in the Farmer kitchen and calling them "these cooking-school messes." Fannie's father, J. Franklin Farmer, was a printer who never could bring himself to adopt modern technology in his small business, and as a result did less and less work as the years went on. Five daughters in all were born to the Farmers—one died in infancy—and although to many families of that time educating four daughters would have been seen as a waste of time and money, the Farmers made every effort to give them as much schooling as possible. Described by Fannie's niece as "Unitarian and bookish," the Farmer family was far from wealthy, but they greatly valued education and would have been considered a genteel household of "brain workers."

Fannie's three sisters became teachers—her sister Cora was the only one of the daughters who married—and Fannie, who was thought to be especially bright, was going to be sent to college. While she was still at Medford High School, however, she came down with what was probably polio. As one of her childhood friends recalled it many years later, she and Fannie had a date to have their tintypes taken but Fannie never showed up. She had fallen when she tried to get out of bed that morning, and had no sensation in her legs. Her family tried bathing them in warm water, and called a local doctor, who thought that Fannie might have ruptured a blood vessel. Fannie was paralyzed and bedridden for months and remained an invalid for several years. Eventually she was able to walk again, although always with a limp. The illness prevented her from finishing high school and it also made her an unlikely candidate for marriage. Until she was well into her twenties it seemed as though she would be wholly dependent upon her parents. She was as bright as ever and had regained enough strength to work, but there were few employments open to a lady who lacked a high-school diploma, and fewer still to one with a limp. She did housework, of course, and even baked cookies to sell, but her contributions to the family income were negligible.

In order to support the family a bit more easily, the Farmers decided to move back to Boston, where they had cousins who wanted to board with them. Over the years the household grew to as many as thirteen, for Fannie and her three sisters all remained at home, and Cora brought in her husband and later had a son. At length Fannie did get a chance to work: she went across the river to Cambridge to be a mother's helper in the Shaw family, where there was a little girl named Marcia. According to at least one apocryphal story, it was while she was employed with the Shaws that she first envisioned the possibilities for the culinary reform with which she is most closely identified. Watching Fannie in the kitchen measuring out "butter the size of an egg" or "a pinch of salt," little Marcia Shaw is supposed to have asked what those expressions meant. At that moment, presumably, standardized level measurements were born. In another version of the same story, Fannie was teaching at the Boston Cooking School when little Marcia Shaw, by then a student at the school, raised her hand to ask the same question. In neither case is Fannie's fateful answer recorded, but she did become interested in cookery when she was employed for the first time, and since the Boston Cooking School did not then require a high-school diploma for admission, the Farmers and the Shaws both urged her to enroll and become a cooking teacher.

Fannie was thirty-one years old when she entered the Boston Cooking School. She had postponed her working life, and the active use of her mind, for over a decade, and she was more than ready to tackle a new world. She did so well at the school that after she completed the normal course she was asked to take the job of assistant to the principal, Carrie Dearborn, a well-liked but chronically frail teacher. Mrs. Dearborn resigned her position in order to take to the lecture circuit in 1893—she died two years later, hailed by Mrs. Lincoln as "the brightest star in the galaxy of homemakers"—and upon her resignation the board of managers quickly chose Fannie as the new principal.

The Boston Cooking School was emerging from some of its more difficult years at the time Miss Farmer took it over. Despite the efforts of the board of managers to run the school in a businesslike fashion after it became incorporated in 1882, they rapidly amassed a large debt when the numbers of pupils did not increase fast enough to keep up with expenses. "There was little knowledge of, and great prejudice against cooking schools," explained the author of a brief official history of the school that appeared in the first issue of *New England Kitchen Magazine*. Equally to the point, perhaps, was the fact that Mrs. Lincoln had resigned in 1885 in order to devote herself full time to the more lucrative work of writing, editing, and lecturing. She had earned an excellent reputation by that time, and the board could find nobody of her standing as a replacement. Ida Maynard, a thoroughly unknown graduate of the school, agreed to take the job, but she was unable to attract many new pupils. At this "trying time," as *New England Kitchen Magazine* put it, "new life was infused into the enterprise." The board managed to raise enough money from wealthy and reform-minded Bostonians to pay off its debt, and then began to advertise aggressively. This new campaign successfully averted the immediate threat, and Carrie Dearborn, who had recently graduated from the school, was chosen to replace the ineffectual Miss Maynard. Mrs. Dearborn, like Mrs. Lincoln before her, became a popular and widely traveled lecturer, and while she was principal a good deal of the original public enthusiasm surrounding the school was restored. Not until the reign of

Miss Farmer, however, did the Boston Cooking School vigorously renew itself and begin to grow.

"Miss F. says if a cook can make a good cream cake, baking-powder biscuit & creamed codfish she can cook almost anything," scribbled one of Miss Farmer's students on the inside cover of her notebook. That sense of absolute conviction toward life in the kitchen was something that all domestic scientists tried to convey, but no one else managed to package it in a style so brisk and effective. Miss Farmer believed that any woman could learn to take charge of what her family ate, and that taking charge did not stop with figuring out the right number of calories. "I for one have no patience with the housewife who always serves her vegetables 'plain boiled,' " she wrote in the *Companion*. "It is impossible to raise cookery above a mere drudgery if one does not put heart and soul into the work; then, and then only, it becomes the most enjoyable of household duties. If reliable recipes are at hand, try them, and you will be repaid a thousand times by family praise." While her colleagues were building up women's role with rationalizations drawn from science, evolution, religion, and patriotism, Miss Farmer looked to simple necessity and the possibility for enjoyment; while others promoted domestic-science education as the only way to transform drudgery, Miss Farmer offered "heart and soul."

Energetic, red-haired, and solidly built, Fannie Farmer was one cooking teacher whom nobody would have called dainty, for she pitched into her work with an unabashed interest in everything to do with eating. She never cared about clothes—her sisters had to urge her to dress up a little when she went out to lecture at women's clubs—and she customarily wore a shoulder-to-ankle white apron and white cap just as her pupils did. Her zeal on the lecture platform was famous: she would mix and measure speedily at her demonstrations and explain each step with directness and clarity. "Our instructors love their work," she told a writer from *Good Housekeeping* who visited the school, "and go into it with the same enthusiasm as if it was music or art." One thing that kept her own enthusiasm up seems to have been a healthy appetite. In contrast to her colleagues she freely described dishes as "tasty," "delicious," "appetizing," and very often "delightful." While other cooks always insisted that their own preferences in food were simple and austere, Fannie Farmer liked to eat and didn't mind saying so. Compared with the boiled white dinners that most cooking schools were producing, Miss Farmer's ideas were distinctly imaginative, and she pursued a taste for novelty and ornament that enthralled her audiences.

Her divergence from the domestic-science movement first became apparent when she revised the classroom text that had been used at the Boston Cooking School since 1884, *Mrs. Lincoln's Boston Cook Book*. Miss Farmer felt that Little, Brown ought to publish the new text, for that very respectable Boston firm had published Louisa May Alcott and other distinguished local authors, and when the manuscript was completed she put on her most ladylike outfit and carried the book to the publisher herself. Cautious and conservative, Little, Brown was unwilling to take a chance on the cookbook but finally drew up an agreement whereby Miss Farmer would be responsible for the publication costs, while Little, Brown simply produced and distributed the book as her agent. Fannie Farmer could have lost heavily with this proposition, for she hadn't much to fall back on if the book proved a financial failure. But with her usual confidence she accepted the risk, and proceeded to make back her original investment and a great deal more. *The Boston Cooking-School Cook Book* appeared in 1896 and quickly sold out its first modest printing of three thousand copies. It was reprinted twice in 1897 and once a year thereafter until 1906, when a revised edition came out. This time the first printing consisted of 20,000 copies, and it, too, was reprinted yearly. When Fannie Farmer died in 1915, over 360,000 copies of the book had been sold, and it was still coming out regularly in printings of 50,000 each.

Several comprehensive and trustworthy cookbooks were on the market in 1896, most notably Mrs. Lincoln's, and many were written by food authorities more famous than Fannie Farmer was at that time. The name of the book certainly accounted for some of its initial appeal, for the Boston Cooking School was known throughout the country, but it wasn't long before the book was better known by its author's name than by its institution's: it became to all who used it the Fannie Farmer cookbook. Mrs. Lincoln, from whose *Boston Cook Book* Miss Farmer had drawn quite liberally, was understandably reluctant to join in the general excitement about the book that was overshadowing her own, and the review in *New England Kitchen Magazine* was grudging. Its anonymous author acknowledged Miss Farmer's popularity as a teacher but urged that "the long procession" of cookbooks and teachers that preceded her not be forgotten. "The book is well arranged in the order which has proved satisfactory in similar works . . ." the reviewer commented, pointedly. "But those who have known anything of the origin and growth of the school will be surprised to find a book with this title containing no mention of Mrs. Lincoln, Miss Maynard and Mrs. Dearborn. For it is to the efforts of those ladies as well as of its present management that the prosperity of the school is due."

Fannie Farmer did help herself, generously and without acknowledgment, to Mrs. Lincoln's work; but she stamped the material with her own personality, or perhaps it is more accurate to say that she drained it carefully of Mrs. Lincoln's. Instead of the comfortable, discursive way in which Mrs. Lincoln addressed her readers, as if she were chatting with each one personally, Fannie Farmer chose a style that was businesslike and to the point. Where Mrs. Lincoln took the role of hostess, making technical information accessible to women by delivering it cozily, Miss Farmer preferred the more distant role of lecturer. On the subject of deep-fat frying, for example, the two cooks made many of the same points in distinctly different voices.

All articles to be fried should be thoroughly dried and slightly warmed [Mrs. Lincoln directed]. If very *moist*, or very *cold*, or *too many* articles be fried at a time, the fat becomes chilled, and the grease soaks into them. Then, as the moisture heats and boils, it causes such a commotion that the fat and water boil over, and there is great danger from the fat taking fire and spreading to your clothing, to say nothing of the trouble of cleaning the stove and floor. For this reason be careful not to let a drop of water, or of condensed steam from another kettle, fall into the hot fat.

Fannie Farmer also warned her readers to dry and warm the food before lowering it into the fat, but her analysis was succinct and she didn't bother with the dangers of household conflagration. "Great care must be taken that too much is not put into the fat at one time, not only because it lowers the temperature of the fat, but because it causes it to bubble and go over the sides of the kettle," she wrote. "It is not fat that boils, but water which fat has removed from food." In a similarly streamlined fashion she reduced to a few terse sentences Mrs. Lincoln's relaxed discussion of the chemical properties of food, and was able to convey the chief necessities for a balanced diet in four paragraphs, while Mrs. Lincoln's thoughts on proper eating habits spanned five pages, touching on the Turks, the Arabs, the Irish, and the "Esquimaux," as well as a number of other examples. Miss Farmer was not the first to base a cookbook on scientific principles, but she was the first to make the information accessible by straight simplification, presenting it without apologies rather than sweetening it to make it palatable for women at home. At a time when writing, especially women's writing for other women, was an exercise in ornamentation, Miss Farmer's direct prose stands out dramatically. *The Boston Cooking-School Cook Book* was written to be consulted, not read, and its aim was to be authoritative, not simply companionable. In tone and function it was the most modern cookbook on the market.

Building and regulating the fire in the stove, arranging the wood nearby for greatest convenience, blackening the stove, sifting the ashes; how to boil, bake, stew, fry, fricassee, and braise; how to bone a bird; how to stir, beat, and whip—Miss Farmer moved quickly through all the basic procedures of the kitchen, but she paused for special emphasis when she arrived at the business of measuring. "Correct measurements are absolutely necessary to insure the best results," she wrote. For her, as for other cooks trained at cooking schools, the popular reliance on luck and guesswork threw a constant shadow over the scientific image of cookery. Exact measurement was the foundation for everything else that happened in the scientific kitchen, although there was not always agreement about how to reach exactitude. Impressionistic quantities like "a handful" or "the size of a hazelnut" plainly were not to be depended upon, and the European practice of weighing ingredients on a kitchen scale, precise though it was, seemed slow and cumbersome to impatient American cooks. Most authorities juggled teacups, salt spoons, and other unwieldy units, employing as much rationality as they could muster, until standard measuring implements came on the market. Half-pint measuring cups first appeared in the mid-1880s and were commonly sold in pairs—one marked in quarters, and the other in thirds. Measuring spoons, and a single cup with two sets of markings, followed not long after; and cooking teachers made them standard equipment in every school. Miss Farmer, who entered the Boston Cooking School just at the time measuring cups were coming into use, was trained to cook with them from the start. Her particular innovation was the refinement known as level measurements, which she promoted forcefully with every recipe she published. Previously even the strictest use of measuring implements retained the old notions of a "rounded" spoonful and a "heaping" cupful. Mrs. Lincoln had been progressive enough to give these terms the most explicit definitions she could come up with—a spoonful was supposed to be "just rounded over, or convex in the same proportion as the spoon is concave," and a "heaping" spoonful or cupful was all that it would hold—and she also noted that "butter the size of an egg" equaled one heaping tablespoonful. To Fannie Farmer it seemed simpler and more rational to dispense with the imagery entirely and call a tablespoonful a level tablespoon, using a knife to level the surface after the spoon had been filled. *"A cupful is measured level,"* she wrote with a rare indulgence in italics. *"A tablespoonful is measured level. A teaspoonful is measured level."* These pronouncements appeared unfailingly in her cookbooks, her magazine articles, and her lectures, finally earning her the epithet the "Mother of Level Measurements."

Miss Farmer's interest in exact measurements went far beyond cups and spoons, however: she liked to specify that strips of pimento used for decoration be cut three-quarters of an inch long and half an inch wide, and she could measure out spices by the grain. Occasionally she directed that vegetables used in salad should be cut "in fancy shapes" or that a sauce should be "seasoned highly," but instructions allowing the cook that much margin for imagination—and hence for error—were the exceptions. Her approach to cooking was above all that of a teacher, and she designed *The Boston Cooking-School Cook Book* to free its readers as much as possible from any moments of hesitation or uncertainty in the kitchen. Exhaustive precision was not a burden to Miss Farmer but a means to speedy work and assured results. The sense of control offered by this emphasis on exactitude, along with the book's greatly simplified introduction to food chemistry, made up a version of scientific cookery that housekeepers found very easy to adopt, whether or not they had any interest in Professor Atwater or any desire to use a dietary computer.

Although she kept information and advice pared to its most comprehensible minimum, Miss Farmer was lavish with the recipes themselves, working out numerous variations and novelties on many of the basic preparations. Sometimes her variations consisted in little more than changing the names and proportions of Mrs. Lincoln's recipes, but she did append a dozen or more new ones in most sections of the book. These were often recipes, or at least names and themes, that she borrowed from some of the fashionable eating places of Boston and New York. Her "Eggs *à la Finnois*"—poached eggs in a tomato sauce—was based on a dish from Delmonico's, and she cooked mushrooms *"à l'Algonquin,"* chicken *"à la Metropole,"* and oysters *"à la Thorndike."* If Mrs. Lincoln gave directions for an omelet and suggested a few different fillings, Fannie Farmer did the same, but couldn't resist adding a border of white sauce. To Mrs. Lincoln's unpretentious salads—in 1884 she was making nothing more elaborate than a chicken salad swathed in mayonnaise, or a salmon salad cupped in a lettuce leaf—Miss Farmer added directions for a tomato jelly molded and trimmed to look like fresh tomatoes; sweetbreads and cucumbers stuffed into cucumber boats; and a variety of decorative arrangements with nuts, cheese, eggs, and diced vegetables. With desserts she was similarly abundant, and she included an entirely new section of recipes for the chafing dish, as well as a chapter on candy.

The unique combination of directness and novelty that marked Miss Farmer's approach to cooking attracted a huge and devoted following. Soon after she became principal, the Boston Cooking School began to outgrow its original home, and the year after the cookbook was published the school had to move to new and larger quarters. The board expressed some fear that the move would throw them back into financial disarray, but when the first pupils showed up at the new building for the opening of the school year, it became clear that increased numbers already justified the move and might soon necessitate another one. In the five years following the publication of the book the size of the normal class doubled, and attendance at Miss Farmer's demonstration lectures grew to over three thousand a year. A second assistant was hired for Miss Farmer, the demand for private lessons increased, aspiring nurses filled eight special classes in invalid cookery, and Miss Farmer lectured regularly to the fourth-year class at Harvard Medical School, as well as keeping up numerous outside speaking engagements. Despite all this activity and her own indisputable success, however, Miss Farmer was getting restless. Perhaps because she had entered the Boston Cooking School relatively late in her life, she was never so definitively influenced by it as were her classmates and colleagues. The school started her on her career, and she reflected its ways and values in her approach to basic cooking, but once she became an authority in her own right, she began to grow away from the school. The Boston Cooking School curriculum was organized to offer the essentials of science and cookery in a short time, especially to women who planned to become classroom teachers rather than cooks. It was not a distinction that most of her colleagues cared to recognize, but Fannie Farmer could see the difference. Training teachers was dull work to her; she much preferred giving private lessons to ladies who came individually to the Boston Cooking School, or sent their cooks, to learn puff paste or lobster Newburg or Baked Alaska. The normal course, she believed, put too much emphasis on scientific theory and not enough on practical work in the kitchen. After Miss Farmer had been there ten years, the Boston Cooking School did set up a course in "plain and fancy cooking," which was, the announcement specified, "designed especially for housekeepers and those *not* intending to teach." Nevertheless, at the end of what must have been a drab school year in 1901—the graduation ceremonies featured a commencement address on "Cold Water" and another on "Hot Water"—Miss Farmer resigned from the school and made plans to open her own. The class of 1902 was the last one she taught, and the class of 1903 was the last in the history of the Boston Cooking School.

The board of managers did not expect the Boston Cooking School to collapse with the departure of Fannie Farmer; on the contrary, they quickly replaced her with one of her assistants, Maria Howard, and signed a new five-year lease for the building. Miss Farmer's final year had been the "most prosperous" the school had ever enjoyed, according to the *Boston Cooking School Magazine*, and the board believed the school would continue to thrive even against competition from the new Miss Farmer's School of Cookery. Evidently they underestimated the powerful attraction of Fannie Farmer's name and culinary style. Miss Farmer's School of Cookery opened in the fall of 1902 and was an immediate success. A few months later the board of the Boston Cooking School announced that it was turning over its lease, its equipment, and even Miss Howard to Simmons College, which had opened just a year earlier. Simmons was founded to train women in practical and technical skills that would enable them to earn their own living, and the department of domestic science was one of the first to be set up. With what the board called the "transfer" of the cooking school to Simmons, the college would now offer cookery using the cooking-school facilities. Although Simmons aimed at training professionals, the board won an agreement that for the next few years the cookery department would offer a one-year course to women planning to be homemakers, as well as a degree program in cookery for teachers. With this assurance—Simmons called it the "diamond-ring course"—the board could retire certain that all the constituents of the Boston Cooking School would be well taken care of under the new management.

Once free from the Boston Cooking School, Fannie Farmer proceeded to set up course work along the lines she liked best, and her inclinations proved to be very profitable. Miss Farmer's School eventually had four kitchens and a staff of ten teachers, and her pupils included young women planning to marry; older women running their own homes; housemaids, cooks, and waitresses sent by their employers to improve their skills; nurses; and even graduates of domestic-science schools, who felt they lacked experience in cooking. Her series of demonstration-lectures for cooks employed in private houses—an audience the Boston Cooking School had been trying and failing to draw for twenty years—attracted well over a hundred cooks each week. The curriculum did feature instruction in the chemistry and physiology of food, but it was kept brief and practical, and illustrated with charts and drawings. There were three general cooking courses: the first beginning with milk toast and creamed chicken and proceeding to other simple dishes; the second more elaborate, arranged for family dinners and entertaining; and the third for more expensive dinners and fancy cookery. A separate course in Chafing-

Dish Cookery, Salads, and Desserts was offered; there was a course in marketing, with visits to the Faneuil Hall market; and there was a crash course—daily for a month—giving the basics in cooking and housekeeping to women who needed to know fast. Later Fannie Farmer opened a summer school for teachers, matrons of institutions, and nurses, as well as housekeepers.

While she was running all these activities and more —for she continued to give demonstration lectures, private lessons, and classes in sickroom cookery—Fannie Farmer was writing columns and assembling menus every month for *The Woman's Home Companion*, working on revisions of *The Boston Cooking-School Cook Book*, and producing five more cookbooks. Despite health problems that became worse as she grew older, especially the trouble with her legs, she worked vigorously at developing recipes, promoting the school, and reaching out to her audience.

> I am enclosing one of each of my demonstration-slips thinking that you may like to file them [she wrote to a former student, who was teaching in Rochester, New York]. [The demonstration slips were printed copies of recipes that were handed out at all lectures.] The butterfly teas were very pretty and well liked. The Russian Eggs made quite a hit. Under separate cover I am mailing a copy of the New Book of Cookery. It will I am sure seem like a visit from an old friend. I trust you will be pleased with the general make up of the book. If you can sell any to your advantage I could send you some in lots of 25 for 1.20 each. I shall always be glad to hear from you and if you have any new recipes that I could use in demonstrations of course they would be much appreciated. Miss Allen has two waitress classes on Monday. One in the a.m. and one in the p.m. Next week we shall be running sixteen hospital classes. sixteen private classes and we start our third marketing class. With the special lessons we are more than busy. I am working to my limit and I am surprised at myself.

Inside this letter Miss Farmer tucked a sketch of the "butterfly tea" she had created—a puff-paste cookie in the shape of a butterfly, decorated painstakingly with chopped nuts, glacéd cherries, angelica, cinnamon, and sugar. The

"Russian Eggs"—on the demonstration slip Miss Farmer jotted, "This came from St. Petersburg"—were boiled, peeled, set into puff-paste cases, and covered with a creamed-mushroom sauce. These were dishes very much in the style for which she was best known in her own time, a style she could only hint at when she wrote *The Boston Cooking-School Cook Book* but that blossomed in the five books that followed: *Chafing Dish Possibilities* (1898), *Food and Cookery for the Sick and Convalescent* (1904), *What to Have for Dinner* (1905), *Catering for Special Occasions* (1911), and *A New Book of Cookery* (1912). The recipes she used in these books, as well as in her lectures and articles, were developed somewhat the way clothing designers develop new fashions—not for their usefulness or even propriety, but for their effect on a chosen constituency. Fannie Farmer knew food very well and could manipulate it adroitly; even more important, she was able to win from her public a fascination with food equal to her own. While her personality in print or on the lecture platform was generally straightforward and without frills, she poured into the recipes themselves all the liveliness and sentiment that were abbreviated in her prose. Most of her scientific colleagues reversed those emphases, presenting themselves to the public with a great deal of warmth and charm but specializing in largely functional food. To be sure, the vogue for encapsulated salads and color-coordinated meals at times drew in even the most sober cooking-school graduate, but Miss Farmer was uniquely talented at putting her education toward the service of delight. When she made croquettes, for example, she was careful to describe each step of the process and to enumerate all the possible causes for failure; but she was also capable of shaping them into chickens and ducklings, with peppercorns for eyes. Discussing the nutritive value of fruits in the *Companion*, she dwelt briefly on their mineral constituents but then went so far as to point out their "delicious flavors," nutritionally useless though that property was. "It is usually agreed that fruits are never better than when served fresh," Miss Farmer acknowledged; nonetheless, the recipes she chose on this occasion ranged far from that ideal, including as they did sautéed pears in chocolate sauce, frozen charlotte glacé made with peach ice cream, fruit soufflé, and melon croquettes. The only raw fruits to show up in this column were covered immediately with sherbet or salad dressing or whipped cream. In a later article she drew attention to the food value in dried fruits, and urged her readers to stuff dried figs with marshmallows and candied cherries, in the interest of their impressive carbohydrate count, before she dutifully wrote a paragraph about stewed prunes. When it came to outright festivity, of course, she had no equal in the domestic-science movement. While she was not the only cooking teacher to turn Valentine's Day into the occasion to demonstrate a pink-and-white repast, few others would have taken the trouble to make the salmon, the Lovers' Sandwiches, and the Heart's-Ache Pudding all in the shape of hearts, or to hide morsels of cream-cheese-and-olives between two walnut halves to make "Cupid's Deceits." On St. Patrick's Day she liked to have everything as green as possible—she even dyed the sauterne that topped a dish of sherbet—and she showed how to tie popcorn balls with green ribbons, upon which she glued "St. Patrick" in letters made of macaroni. "For a real Christmas dessert Parisian doll ice cream takes the banner for me this year," she wrote once in the *Companion*, evincing more excitement than she usually did in print. "I found the conceit in New York this summer, but I hope by the holiday season it will make many an eye twinkle at the Christmas dinner." The dessert that had aroused her interest so was a simple dish of ice cream covered with crushed macaroons. Placed over each dish, however, was a four-inch wooden doll dressed in an intricate red-and-green crepe-paper outfit; and it was Miss Farmer's minutely detailed directions for the outfit that constituted the "recipe."

In search of ideas like these, Fannie Farmer made a practice of visiting the leading restaurants in Boston and New York, often accompanied by her parents. At the table they would order as many different things as they could, and Miss Farmer would ponder an unfamiliar sauce all through the meal if she couldn't figure out what was in it. Sometimes she would have to ask the chef for the recipe, and if he was not willing to reveal it, she would carry away a bit of the food on her calling card, to be analyzed later at the school. At home she experimented constantly with new recipes and variations, for with her books, magazine columns, and lectures to fill she always needed fresh ideas. "Couldn't it be better?" she would prod her family and students as they tasted. A flair for novelty was an important part of her appeal, and she flogged her imagination for new ways, new ingredients, and new combinations.

Fannie Farmer often said that the work she was proudest of was *Food and Cookery for the Sick and Convalescent*, a book she dedicated lovingly to her mother. From personal experience she knew very well what it was like to be bedridden and restricted for long periods of time, and how much the quality of nursing affected the mood of the invalid. At Miss Farmer's School her courses in sick-room cookery were advertised as the "specialty of the school." When the context was diet and medical practice, she plainly enjoyed dwelling a bit on the scientific theories that she skimmed in her other work. In *Food and Cookery* she discussed nutrition, the variables in the digestive process, and the special requirements of infants and children with more substance and spirit than those topics received anywhere else in her writing. Her sensitivity to the emotional state of the patient was especially acute. "Never serve a patient custard scooped out from a large pudding dish," she advised in a lecture at the Adams Nervine Asylum, a hospital specializing in "nervous" disorders, which was located in suburban Jamaica Plain. "He wants to feel that he is being particularly looked out for, and the individual custard suits him. Please your patient whenever you can. No matter how scientific a doctor may be, if he is brusque he doesn't please, and a pleasing personality is a success no matter what the pursuit."

Miss Farmer did not believe that patients should be allowed to indulge their cravings or even that they should be consulted about the menu, since she thought disease imposed a certain perversion on the appetite. Nor did she feel it was good practice to discuss matters of diet where the invalid could hear. In preparing the sickroom tray, however, there were six considerations for the cook to keep in mind, and Miss Farmer listed them in order of importance: appealing to the sight, appealing to the taste, serving the food at the proper temperature, the digestibility of the meal, its nutritive value, and its cost. Only a cooking teacher who understood illness could have ranked these points as she did. Most of Miss Farmer's colleagues would have chosen the opposite order, but her commitment to spurring the appetite with eye-catching food was even greater in the sickroom than it was at the dinner table. No matter how simple or bland the meal might be, the bread could be cut into the shape of hearts; the ice cream served in a flower pot with a daisy stuck into it; the blancmange molded in an egg cup and garnished with a candied cherry; and the creamed peas spooned into a croustade cut from bread, with a leaf of parsley at the corner. Gelatin, the staple of the sickroom, lent itself to a great many decorative poses. Orange jelly could be jelled, albeit with some difficulty, inside a scooped-out orange; plain gelatin made with sugar and egg white could be cut to look like marshmallows. And wine jelly could be molded in a whiskey glass until firm, leaving aside two tablespoonfuls of the liquid jelly. These should be beaten until white and frothy, then set atop the molded jelly. "It will suggest a freshly drawn glass of beer," Miss Farmer wrote hopefully.

After she reached her mid-fifties Miss Farmer's own health began to fail seriously, and she once again lost the use of her legs. For the last two years of her life she lectured from a wheelchair. During this time she remained as active as she could—when she traveled she would call ahead to be met with a wheelchair—and she worked at a good pace right up until her death. On December 30, 1914, she presented a lecture on what would be her last dinner party menu, and it made an impressive and wholly characteristic conclusion to her work in fancy cookery. The main course was veal olives—pieces of veal wrapped in bacon—but the attention-getter was their escort: a serving of Thorndike potatoes, which were potatoes and bananas mashed together, stuffed into banana skins, sprinkled with parmesan, and broiled. A Tango Salad came next—avocados cut to look like horseshoes with bits of truffle to represent the nails. The centers were filled with orange sections, and the whole covered with a cooked dressing made of condensed milk, whipped cream, and orange juice. To serve alongside the salad Miss Farmer fried up some Pimento and Cheese Fritters, which she made by inserting a slice of American cheese into a canned pimento, dredging it with flour, and sautéing until the cheese began to melt. Dessert was a frozen Pineapple Bombe, in which pineapple sherbet was used to line a mold that was then filled with custard and candied fruit. Miss Farmer described it to her audience as a "German favorite." A week later she presented a lecture on Breakfast and Sandwich Breads, but she was becoming ill at about that time and was taken to the hospital a few days later. She never gave the next week's demonstration, which was to have been on one of her favorite subjects—cake and frosting. On Friday, January 15, 1915, she died at the hospital. Her illness was called "neuritis" at the time, but later diagnosis cited arteriosclerosis. The *Boston Evening Transcript* ran her obituary on the front page; and she was buried in Mount Auburn Cemetery—perhaps a choice made by her mother, for this was the accepted resting place for true Bostonians.

As the most successful by far of the cooking-school cooks, Fannie Farmer died rich. Besides investing carefully in utilities, railroads, and a chocolate company, along with other certainties, she distributed her savings among nineteen different bank accounts. She also owned her old home in Medford, as well as a parcel of land in Harvard, Massachusetts, where she had started to build a country house for her family. With the school and the copyrights to her books, Miss Farmer's estate came to nearly $200,000. At the time of her death, the current edition of *The Boston Cooking-School Cook Book* had been revised to incorporate

A New Book of Cookery, so the lavish culinary style that made her distinctive was at last fully represented in the plain-spoken book that made her famous.

Fannie Farmer's climb up the American ladder from mere gentility to visible wealth made a feminine variation on the usual Horatio Alger story, and one that was absorbed via her recipes in millions of kitchens. The women who responded so overwhelmingly to Miss Farmer's way of cooking were part of the country's most open-bordered social class, in which education and correct living were expected to lead straight up. The salads, desserts, and chafing-dish items in honor of which she set up a special course at Miss Farmer's School were touchstones in the realm of socially ambitious cookery, for many of them took more time than skill, and qualified, literally, as conspicuous consumption. Miss Farmer's reliable instructions made it possible for even the least sophisticated housekeeper to serve *Bombe de Fillets de Fish à la Richelieu* if she could afford the ingredients, and if she couldn't, Fannie Farmer had directions for placing a paper frill on pork chops and serving them in nests of mashed potato. Here was a way of cooking that put high-class food within the reach of ordinary housekeepers and made up-to-date novelties accessible as well—all in the context of progress. When Fannie Farmer at last set down her measuring spoons and gave in to her final illness, she left behind a kitchen she had helped, crucially, to redirect toward social homogeneity and American cheese..

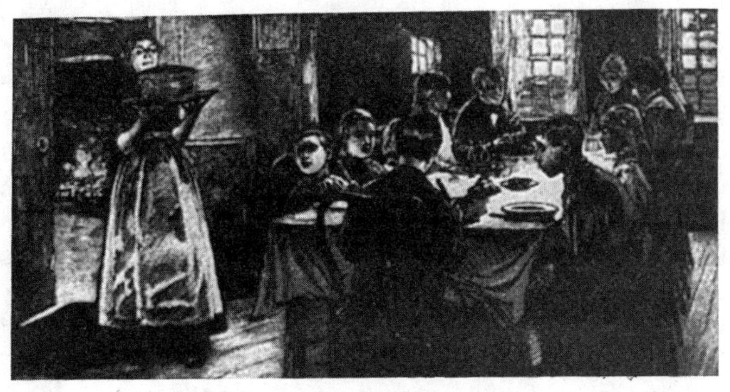

Six

Whoever Knew a Dyspeptic to Be a Christian?

In the spring of 1897 a yellow-and-violet dinner was prepared and served by a class of cooking students in Morganza, Pennsylvania. Yellow roses and violets were set on the table, yellow tissue-paper cups were filled with candied orange peel, and each portion of orange sherbet was packed inside an orange skin. Cooking-school specialties such as cream of asparagus soup and halibut with potato balls were offered to an appreciative delegation of ladies, and the students, who were uniformed in blue dresses and white baker's caps, received many compliments. The occasion was a cooking-school commencement like many others—indeed, the only respect in which it differed from similar ceremonies in Boston and Philadelphia was that this cooking course was housed in a reform school and the cooks were young delinquents.

Cooking-school soups and custards would hardly have been deemed worthy of the attention they received during this era if they had not been viewed as important spurs to moral uplift. "Ah!" wrote a Michigan clubwoman, "it sometimes seems a wicked mockery to implore divine deliverance from the drink evil and the social evil while we forget that so many kitchens of the land are sowing seeds which the saloon and the brothel stand ready to cultivate. . . . To dignify the function of the humble kitchen until it becomes in the estimation of every woman a laboratory wherein God permits her to aid in fashioning human souls, is worthy of strenuous endeavor." This analysis, coming at a time of increasingly visible poverty with its attendant misery, alcoholism, prostitution, and disease, was accepted in many reform circles; within the domestic-science movement it was a founding creed. "It is an interesting fact," commented Sarah Tyson Rorer, "that a well-fed man was never behind the bars. . . . Whoever knew a dyspeptic to be a Christian?" Feeding the poor had long been a standard act of charity, but in the view of domestic scientists its traditional format—a photo spread in *The Woman's Home Companion* entitled "The Splendid Christmas Charities of the Great Cities" showed "pickaninnies" receiving leftover eggnog—lacked substance and responsibility. They didn't want to simply feed the poor, they wanted to rebuild the poor, and most cooking schools were established originally in that visionary frame of mind, to spread what was known as the "gospel of good cooking" among the kitchens of the ignorant. Maria Parloa, who did some of the earliest teaching of cookery in New England in the 1870s, hoped that in time every village would have its own cooking school for young girls. "Schools like these," she prophesied, "would bring down the percentage of criminals and paupers, for dirty homes and improper food fill our prisons and almshouses with drunkards and criminals."

The sense of mission that fueled the domestic-science movement and gave it much of its most rousing public vocabulary reflected a safe and sturdy identity traditional among American women activists. Women had long been the guardians of religion in American life: they were the churchgoers; they wrote the tracts and Bible stories; they taught the Sunday schools; they were converted dramatically and in immense numbers; and they served to embody piety within the family and in the community. Every woman was empowered to think of herself as a missionary, assigned to her own household, and one of the few respectable outlets for an independent woman with more energy than her house could contain was real missionary work, on the frontier or in foreign countries. This activity in the spiritual realm offered a useful and appropriate model for reform work on a worldly level. Organized benevolence had first appeared in American society toward the end of the eighteenth century, when sewing circles and other informal women's gatherings turned their conversation and then their capabilities to the plight of poor widows, homeless children, and fallen women. Later, the abolition and temperance movements were significantly driven forward by women, and throughout the nineteenth century small and large projects for moral regeneration flourished on women's philanthropy. As speakers, as teachers, as organizers, and as enthusiastic volunteers in the service of numerous causes, women took on the stance and the rhetoric of those doing the Lord's work.

Perfect housekeeping, of course, was easier than most reforms to conflate with perfect holiness, since the two had long been indistinguishable. "Jane, making a pudding well, sweeping a floor spotlessly, turning the crooked picture on the wall straight . . . performing each and every one of the homely drudgeries of the very homely life . . . is fitting herself for a pure, holy, esthetic heaven . . ." mused the author of a typical sketch called, with gentle irony, "A Wasted Life." When domestic scientists took over the realm of the old domestic moralists, they retained these protective haloes and simply realigned them somewhat. Science and morality became partners, buoyed up by the language and zeal of divine sanction. "If we do our work well," a cooking teacher told her colleagues at the Cooking Teachers' League, "we are the high priestesses of the new religion of right living."

One of the earliest efforts to integrate scientific thinking into moral housekeeping was carried out by Mary

Peabody Mann, who published *Christianity in the Kitchen* in 1857, shortly after her husband, Horace Mann, became the first president of Antioch College. An educator herself, and one who made a number of forward-looking observations on the moral development of children, Mrs. Mann devoted the greatest part of her considerable energies to her husband's work, assisting him at the college and in his research. After his death she promptly wrote his biography and edited his papers, producing a three-volume work in short time. She then produced several more books, including a novel that she completed just before her own death. While her husband was alive, however, Mrs. Mann published only her study of food and righteousness, which she subtitled "A Physiological Cookbook." Her aim was to bring science and physiology into a new "gospel of the body," and to impress upon her readers the benefits of dining in accordance with reason and conscience, rather than gross self-indulgence.

> Compounds like wedding cake, suet plum-puddings, and rich turtle soup, are masses of indigestible material, which never should find their way to any Christian table [she directed]. It looks ominous to see a bridal party celebrating nuptials by taking poison. Although some persons may seem to eat these criminal preparations with present impunity, yet a book of reckoning is kept for the offences of the stomach, as well as for those of the heart, and this is one of the deeds done in the body, for which the doer will be called to account.

Mrs. Mann was writing before most of the advances in nutritional research had been made or publicized in America, but she delved into the major studies that were available. Anticipating many of the themes promoted by scientific cooks forty years later, she spoke out strongly for the efficacy of cream and the saving powers of rice, and she judged foods according to digestion timetables. "Chemical analysis should be the guide for the cookery book," she urged, and looked forward gladly to the day when a laboratory microscope would be standard equipment in every kitchen.

Mrs. Mann's ability to associate scientific cookery with moral cookery, and to use it with propriety as a vehicle for her own intellectual activity, marked her as a woman ahead of her time. After the Civil War, when the domestic-science movement came into prominence, the active, independent women who liked to travel around the country lecturing on the chemistry of bread and the digestibility of soup regularly described themselves as responding, like obedient missionaries, to "a call" from a university, or moving to a new city to take up "the work." In their audiences, and among their pupils, were middle-class women for whom church and charity still provided the most honorable opportunities to get out of the house. Domestic science promised elements of both, and offered a vivid intellectual challenge as well. The women who found their heart's cause in the new movement, whether they were professionals or pupils, seized it with all the energy they had, and wielded it in every direction open to them.

Their immediate target was the poor. The living conditions suffered by immigrants, low-paid workers, and the unemployed had been well publicized since the Civil War, and this wretched home life became immensely interesting to reformers who considered themselves progressive. The philanthropists, the charity workers, the missionaries, and others who made a business of attending to blacks and immigrants thought of them as "foreigners," inadequately civilized, and not yet equipped for the modern world. Reformers did want to relieve suffering, but many felt they could be most efficacious by prodding their charges toward a higher realm of humanity. To them, slum dwellers appeared rather like children, clinging willfully to their bad food, slovenly habits, and foolish predilections. In consonance with this prevailing attitude, domestic scientists viewed the poor and working classes with a mixture of pity and impatience. Plainly it was imperative to reduce the miseries that accrued from bad housing and treacherous working conditions, but unless these families were willing to properly adjust their eating habits, no change in their condition seemed possible.

Nothing stung the domestic scientists more than the thought of a family relying on flimsy, store-bought bread, cheap pastry, and strong tea for their calories. In a collection of garish reports from city slums entitled *Darkness and Daylight, or, Lights and Shadows of New York Life*, the reformer Helen Campbell related in despair how one Irish tenement dweller prepared a meal for her children. " 'Poor folks can't have much roastin' nor fine doin's,' " she quoted "Norah" as saying. " 'Sometimes we has mate, but not often, God knows.' " A piece of "coarse beef" was set in a frying pan with a lump of fat and cooked until it was black and smoking, Mrs. Campbell wrote, while a pot of "rank" tea boiled and Norah cut up a loaf of bread—"its peculiar white color indicating plainly what share alum had had in making the lightness to which she called my attention." As Norah served her "pale-faced and slender" children, Mrs. Campbell left their flat in frustration. "Fried boot-heel would have been as nourishing and as toothsome as that steak, and boiled boot-heel as desirable as and far less harmful a drink than the tea," she wrote, "yet any word of suggestion would have roused the quick Irish temper to fever-heat.

" 'It's Norah can cook equal to yerself,' she once exclaimed to me with pride. . . ."

Trying to be modern and constructive in their approach to people like Norah, domestic scientists took their cue from advocates of the new "scientific charity," reformers who were imposing system and rationality upon traditional female benevolence just as domestic scientists were redefining traditional female work. Proponents of scientific charity disparaged the old-fashioned way of helping families in trouble—handing out food to beggars at the back door, for example, or giving money to every raggedly dressed woman with a baby and a convincing plea. The modern approach was to replace this unthinking and uncontrolled almsgiving with assistance on an organized basis. All requests for help in a city or neighborhood would be channeled to a central office and then investigated individually by charity workers. By making what were called "friendly visits" to each family, a worker could check on the general condition of the home, the family's food and clothing, the degree of cleanliness maintained, whether the husband was trying in earnest to support the family, and whether there was evidence of alcoholism. After this information was assembled, a judgment would be made at the central office as to whether assistance was going to be truly useful or whether it would simply encourage the family to rely on outsiders. Friendly visitors viewed the poor as either "deserving"—people who had been more or less accidentally tumbled into their degrading circumstances and were striving to meet them with dignity—or "undeserving"—those who seemed to be contented or at least passive about their own disgrace.

Reformers who actually lived among the poor interpreted their problems differently. In 1889 Jane Addams and Ellen Starr opened Chicago's Hull-House, the nation's first settlement house, and within two decades reformers inspired by their example had established similar centers in slums throughout the country. The residents at the most active settlement houses were working for social and political reforms in their neighborhoods and cities, as well as offering classes, child care, meeting places, and a myriad of other services for the community. At Hull-House the residents supported strikers, backed reform political candidates, investigated slums and sweatshops, and organized local civic associations. "Settlement workers are likely to say that the sufferings of the poor are due to conditions over which the poor have no control," warned Mary Richmond, one of the leaders in the scientific charity movement, in a handbook called *Friendly Visiting Among the Poor*. She advised friendly visitors to remain aware of bad industrial conditions and defective laws and policies, but never to lose sight of the central importance of human character in the problem of poverty. The rich, she explained, owed justice as well as mercy to the poor, and the poor were in turn "masters of their fate," much more so than some reformers understood. "A political writer has said that formerly, when our forefathers became dissatisfied, they pushed farther into the wilderness, but that now, if anything goes wrong, we run howling to Washington, asking special legislation for our troubles," she added ruefully. ". . . In so far as our charitable work affects it, let us see to it that we do our part in restoring a tone of sturdy self-reliance and independence to the Commonwealth."

As it happened, Helen Campbell came across a widow during her investigations who perfectly exemplified this kind of self-reliance. An Irish woman who had once known better times, she was forced to care for herself and her daughter on eighty-five cents a day. This she managed to do by keeping careful accounts and making a great deal of cabbage soup, and she maintained a very respectable home in a tenement "inhabited chiefly by the better class of Irish." The courageous widow, whom Mrs. Campbell quoted admiringly without adding a trace of the brogue that identified Norah, displayed a thrift and resourcefulness that wiped out all evidence of her normally degrading nationality. In every sense except income, the widow deserved a place in the middle class. According to Mrs. Campbell, the cabbage soup had as much to do with the woman's exemplary success as anything else. "Philanthropists may urge what reforms they will,—less crowding, purer air, better sanitary regulations; but this question of food underlies all," she stressed. "Food easily procured, sufficiently palatable to ensure no dissatisfaction and demanding no ingenuity of preparation, would seem the ideal diet of the poor, if they could be made to adopt it."

The first attempt by an American to create such an ideal diet for the poor was made by Juliet Corson, the superintendent of the New York Cooking School. A frail young woman of genteel background, Miss Corson had been making a modest career writing on various literary and artistic topics when the women's reform organization to which she belonged asked her to teach their cooking class for workingmen's wives and daughters. She was not an experienced cook, but when she was invited to lecture on the subject she quickly did some research and delivered a series of talks that was very well received. In 1876 she opened what became the New York Cooking School in her own home in response to a request from several members of the organization who were interested in classes for themselves. Within a year she was teaching simple and elaborate cookery to women of all social classes; but economical cookery for the poor remained her culinary specialty, and she was a frequent guest instructor at missions, orphanages, and industrial training schools. In 1877, during a time of massive labor turmoil and strikes, she wrote a booklet called *Fifteen Cent Dinners for Workingmen's Families*. When no charitable organization could be persuaded to publish it, she had it printed at her own expense and distributed it free. "All persons are cautioned not to pay for this book," she inscribed in the front of the book. "This edition of 50,000 copies is published for free circulation only." Miss Corson advertised her book widely, and up to two hundred people a day would call at her house for a copy. According to a respectful biographical sketch of Miss Corson, published in her lifetime, she commonly received letters of request from a notably deserving class of poor people: "Please send me a book for people of refinement and education reduced almost to starvation. God will reward you tenfold . . ."; "I feel as if one of your little books would bring light and happiness into my home again . . ."; "I work in a shop where we are getting 80 cents to $1.44 a day. . . . If any person with an intelligent eye would walk through our shops and take notice of our lean, haggard, worn-out faces and bodies, he would come to the conclusion we need some advice." Charities helped to distribute the book—members of the Woman's Education Association in Boston passed out five hundred copies—and newspapers wrote it up approvingly. In the midst of its success Miss Corson's reputation was attacked, according to a report in *Harper's New Monthly*, by "political demagogues and socialists, who inflamed the minds of the workingmen by assuring them that the author was in league with the capitalists, and if they listened to her, and learned how to live better on less money, employers would immediately reduce their wages." The disturbance died down quickly enough, however. "Miss Corson's free lectures are now attended by large and respectful audiences of this class," the magazine concluded.

Miss Corson was unlikely to have been motivated by a desire to lower the wages of workingmen. She had been turned out of her own comfortable home by a stepmother who felt that the young woman should be supporting herself, and for a time she lived on four dollars a week, which she earned from working in a library. Despite the success she enjoyed later as an author and a teacher, Miss Corson was never wealthy, and by the time of her final illness a collection had to be taken among her colleagues to raise funds for her support and medical care. As an educated woman of good background, Juliet Corson would not have been considered poor even when she had no money, but she understood better than many of her colleagues what it meant to live within tight margins. "I hope to live to see the time when workingmen can earn enough to supply all their wants," Miss Corson wrote. "Until then my duty is to show them how to make the best of what they have. And I hold that in doing so I am proving myself a better friend to them than those who try to make them still more discontented with the lot that is already almost too hard to bear."

While the menus in *Fifteen Cent Dinners* were overwhelmingly plain, Miss Corson's awareness of the pleasure that was owed even to the poor at dinner was livelier than many of her colleagues would have thought necessary. A typical day's menu devised by Miss Corson listed broth and bread for breakfast, mutton and turnips for dinner, and barley boiled in broth for supper. At the same time, however, she gave more explicit attention to the imaginative use of herbs and spices than could be found in many upper-class cookbooks, pointing out that her readers could grow tarragon, basil, thyme, mint, and other herbs easily and inexpensively. Tinctures of lemon, orange, and vanilla preserved in alcohol could be made cheaply, too, she noted, and she described how to prepare a pint of tarragon vinegar for six cents. Although she refused to give recipes for pies and cakes ("They are the bane of American Cookery; they are expensive and unhealthy"), she did find she could "safely recommend" several puddings made with rice or suet. Occasionally Miss Corson could not disguise her own distaste for some of the food she suggested for her readers, notably when she was giving directions for choosing second-rate meat. These cuts, she assured her readers, constituted "cheap and good food," but her adjectives belied this message. The less expensive beef, she wrote with distaste, was "rough," "gristly," "tough to the touch." Cheap lamb could be identified by its "coarser" appearance; the poorest pork was "coarse-grained" and "discoloured." In better faith she was able to urge workingmen and their families to try lentils and macaroni, foods she described as unfamiliar to them but which would supply a little variety at low cost.

One reason for Miss Corson's emphasis on making the workingmen's dinners "savory and nutritious" as well as inexpensive was the widespread belief that there was a highly significant connection between bad cooking and the urge for alcohol. Drunkenness was devastating the homes of the poor and working classes in this era, and reformers were certain that alcoholism could be traced directly to hunger. "What you need when you crave liquor is a good, warm meal," Miss Corson advised workingmen, and she warned their wives that a sodden mess of unappealing food "sends the man to the liquor shop for consolation." As the *Boston Cooking School Magazine* saw it: "The laborer who leaves home in the early morning, after an ill-cooked breakfast, and carries in his basket soggy bread and tough meat for his luncheon, is apt to return at night tired and cross; not unfrequently he tries, *en route*, to cure his discomfort at a neighboring saloon, especially if he knows he will find his dinner as uninviting as were his breakfast and luncheon." In San Francisco a cooking teacher was delighted when she asked her pupils to describe the benefits of cooking lessons, for a "serious, sweet-faced" little girl promptly explained that " 'if we knew how to cook lots of nice things, and what kinds of foods were "healthy," the men and boys would like to stay home more, and not go to saloons so much.' " In this assumption domestic scientists and their pupils were joined by members of the flourishing temperance movement and many other social activists, including the urban reformer Jacob Riis, who told a Boston audience that the best way to teach temperance in a tenement house was " 'a cooking school, slapped down right there in the middle of the block.' " Even Professor Atwater, the food chemist, attributed drunkenness among wage earners to " 'poor food and unattractive home tables,' " noting that in some homes he had investigated, proper family meals were unheard of, and food was simply left on a bare table for family members to grab when they could.

In the decades following the publication of *Fifteen Cent Dinners*, Miss Corson and her colleagues steadily increased their faith in the moral and social beneficence of scientific cookery and housekeeping. Speaking to an audience of Christian women's organizations, Miss Corson urged them to support cooking schools not only because "a man is what his food makes him" but because practical education of this sort would be welcomed by the people themselves. "These ideas are by no means radical," she assured her audience; "it is already acknowledged that the result of such education is to counteract discomfort and discontent among all social classes." During these years the country underwent many periods of severe economic stress culminating in the crash of 1893, wage cuts and unemployment brought about bitter protests and strikes, and the specter of a socialist revolution began to loom in the public imagination. Domestic scientists, along with their allies in other reform movements, identified the well-run home as the most powerful guardian of civil peace. "The man who has such a home is not going to join in rash movements of any kind, or in any way jeopardize the possession of that home," wrote the author of an article called "The Home and the Labor Problem." "Has any one ever heard of a strike among any class of laborers in Philadelphia?" she demanded. "I have not. In no other city in the world, perhaps, are found such attractive and comfortable homes for laborers as there." Sarah Tyson Rorer, writing in *Household News* in 1893, just after the bloody Homestead strike and shortly before the even bloodier Pullman strike, placed the blame for these troubles directly upon the workmen's food. "Many of the so-called strikers would strike no matter how much work they had on hand," she argued. "They are illy fed. Not from lack of money, but from *lack of knowledge*. Poor things, how are they to find out the best food to sustain their needs? . . . I verily believe if the rigid instructions for food and feeding were implanted in the minds of our girls during their early school days, the labor element would not be such discontented individuals."

Few of her colleagues spoke out as bluntly as Mrs. Rorer on controversial labor issues, but most of them shared her belief in the political efficacy of dinner. "I am fully persuaded . . ." announced an Omaha clubwoman at a meeting, "that by using every possible means to educate the wives and daughters of working men to be more intelligent home makers, we can do more towards the solution of the labor problem than all the anarchists, the communists, the socialists or even the labor organizations . . . have ever been able to do."

With these national considerations to bolster their charitable sympathies, reformers rapidly established cooking classes in settlement houses, YWCAs, girls' clubs, city missions, juvenile reformatories, and other sites where it seemed likely that they might find the girls and women who would be keeping house for the country's work force. Satisfying numbers of pupils turned up in some cases—the ladies running the Boston Cooking School were proud of the hundreds who were attracted to the school's branch in Boston's Italian district—but by far the best opportunity to install the principles of scientific cookery on a grand scale was offered by the public schools. Many school systems at this time were adding courses in manual training to the elementary and high-school curricula, partly in order to counter what some educators saw as the untoward number of students planning to find work in offices and the professions. "It has long been a matter of deep regret and even of apprehension that a large proportion of our young people are growing up with a positive distaste for manual labor," reported a New York school committee studying the problem, and added, "With an ever-increasing number almost any other form of occupation is preferred." Formal course work in manual training, they hoped, would lend dignity and stature to industrial occupations and help to provide the nation with disciplined, dedicated workers for its expanding industries. The same theory could be applied nicely to domestic science—"Our young women, ignorant of the value of home training, persist in fitting themselves for business rather than for household life," complained the president of the National Household Economic Association —and it quickly took its place as the standard female counterpart to industrial education. Once lodged in the public-school system, in fact, domestic science was lodged in American life. Cooking-school graduates found plentiful job opportunities in the public schools, and they planted the ideals of scientific cookery wherever they settled.

Many public-school cookery courses were modeled on the prototype set up in Boston in 1885, when a group of women activists headed by the philanthropist Mary Hemenway first equipped a central practice kitchen for the girls of five city schools. School Kitchen No. 1—so named with a flourish because it was "the first in the city, the first in the country"—attracted a tremendous amount of attention throughout the country. According to an account of the project written by the principal of one of the schools involved, nearly two thousand visitors showed up at the kitchen in its first six years of operation, hoping to watch the girls cooking, to draw diagrams of the arrangements, and to observe the teaching methods. The girls, wearing white aprons and white caps, worked from a special text prepared by Mrs. Lincoln, *The Boston School Kitchen Text-Book*. At the conclusion of one term they cooked and served a dinner to members of the school board, school personnel from other cities, and "prominent educators from various walks in life," as the principal described them. The dinner, which included six formal courses of soup, fish, roast, salad, pudding, and coffee, was assembled for only $1.86, and after the guests had eaten what was assumed to be their fill, the girls dined satisfactorily on the leftovers. It marked, the principal said, "a new revelation in public school instruction: the school kitchen was an established fact." After three years of the experiment, which had been entirely funded by Mrs. Hemenway, the Boston school board agreed to take on the expense, and School Kitchens Nos. 2, 3, 4, 5, 6, and 7 opened quickly in one neighborhood after another.

Like the organizers of the Boston Cooking School, the women who set up School Kitchen No. 1 had to decide what was best to do with the food that the pupils would cook. Simply to let them eat it would have been a distinctly luxurious solution, and more important, one that taught no real lesson. It was finally ruled that the girls would be allowed at least one free taste of everything made, in order that they might learn the correct flavor of each dish, and then at the end of the class they would be permitted to buy, at cost, the food they had cooked. In this way the stews and custards prepared at school would find their way to the girls' homes, which was one of the major goals of the experiment. In addition, the pupils were supposed to take the recipes home with them and cook the same dishes for their families, receiving academic credit for the meals they cooked in their own kitchens. After six years the principal estimated that 1,600 girls had cooked 152,621 dishes at home. "Skilled cookery was thus introduced into many homes, and a new order of living inaugurated in a portion of the community," he attested.

The great challenge for domestic scientists involved in public-school cookery was to impress its academic credibility upon those who still believed that cookery belonged at home, and not in a serious school curriculum. Some parents complained that the work was menial and that their daughters were being taught to be servants, and others believed the girls simply cooked extravagant dishes on fancy equipment and that the whole enterprise was frivolous. "It is amusing and at the same time rather trying to find what curious ideas many people have of the public school work," wrote a Boston cooking teacher. "It almost seems as though the majority think that the time given is merely spent in learning to cook all sorts and kinds of dishes." Domestic scientists constantly emphasized that they were teaching "food principles," not just making pies and cakes, and that the girls were learning essential processes of nutrition and digestion that every woman had a responsibility to understand. They preferred to call the school kitchen a "cooking laboratory" and they fought hard to avert what one school system saw as "the very natural danger of putting teachers into our schools who were simply experts in the practice of cookery. . . ." The way to ensure respect for cookery, it seemed to them, was to work at a strict intellectual distance from food and kitchens, except when pupils were actually cooking. Anna Barrows, one of the most thoroughly pedagogical of the scientific cooks and a strong supporter of public-school cookery—in 1900 she became one of the first women elected to the Boston school board—argued that cooking lessons should be understood as the practical application of physics, chemistry, physiology, and botany. Arithmetic certainly entered into many cooking lessons, she noted, and even English could be taught in the cookery class, for pupils learned as much about language from copying recipes as from copying poetry. The difference between "one tablespoonful of butter melted" and "one tablespoonful of melted butter," Miss Barrows pointed out, constituted in itself a valuable lesson on the importance of word order in a sentence. While she did not expect or even want expert cooks to emerge from a year's course work at one of the school kitchens, Miss Barrows did foresee a new generation of housekeepers who would begin their married lives armed with more knowledge than their mothers had at the start, and a larger respect for the kitchen.

Along with other public-school cookery teachers Anna Barrows believed that manual training and domestic science would act, in the words of a Boston educator, as an "antidote" for class differences. Public schools by definition drew children from widely disparate backgrounds, and one mandate of the school kitchen was to unite all its pupils under a single ideal of domesticity. Like the miscreants of Morganza, Pennsylvania, the girls who participated in these cooking classes were expected to absorb from their instruction a certain moral gentility as well as new habits in the kitchen. "One incidental part of the work the girls enjoy very much, and that is to read what men of culture have thought about cooking and household duties," noted a Boston cooking teacher. "They are surprised and pleased to learn that John Ruskin, Theodore Parker, Nathaniel Hawthorne, George Herbert, and others speak of these things in the highest terms of praise." In this classroom a couplet from Herbert's well-loved comment on housework—"A servant by this clause/Makes drudgery divine/Who sweeps a room as for thy laws,/Makes that an th'action fine"—was permanently affixed to the blackboard. Charity workers had long believed that the surest way to rescue young girls from the evil influences of the shops and streets was to establish in them a deep respect for cooking and housework. According to a Boston schoolmaster, the disorderly girls in his charge did become "humanized and refined" from their experience in cooking class. In another city, the success of the domestic science course was gauged from the opposite perspective: the "dainty daughters" of the local aristocracy had turned into eager students of cooking and cleaning, despite their mothers' initial horror at the idea of their children engaging in servants' work. A kind of democratic leveling was believed possible in the school kitchen, where the great rules and responsibilities that lay behind the perfect boiling of an egg were equally pertinent to females of all social classes. "Our little girl is wonderfully interested in the bacteria of the dishcloth, and the ice box, and the garbage pail, and when she becomes mistress of a home these things will receive her attention as well as the parlor, library, and music room," reported the supervisor of cookery in the New York City school system, describing the typical "little housekeeper" produced in the schools. "If John can not afford to give her all these rooms, she has been trained to know that she can be just as happy if she must make one room answer the three purposes, and besides, being an American, she has this thought to comfort her, that under this glorious Government her thrift and economy may help to place her husband among the millionaires."

While the chance to economize their way to aristocracy may indeed have comforted a few wives, the surest "antidote" to social and economic distinctions was the prominent example of a middle class. The ideal home life that was promoted by domestic scientists was defined not by wealth or even occupation but by correct habits and sensibilities. Certain signs of respectability were available to everyone, presumably, and when they were achieved they lent a uniform measure of dignity regardless of income. At the New York Cooking School, where separate courses were set up for "ladies" and for the daughters of "artisans," Juliet Corson used to warn the students in the artisans' course to pour the gravy carefully on the meat "without slopping it over the dish," a nicety she felt no need to state in the ladies' course. Cleanliness, order, decorum; a visible refinement; a cultivated intelligence—these features of what domestic scientists called "right living" comprised a standard of domesticity they hoped to instill everywhere in American society, although they were aware that some populations would require a more thorough overhaul than others. With scientific cookery as the chief means—as well as much of the goal—they hoped to regulate the messy sprawl of American society and to filter out the most unsettling aspects of its diversity. Writing in *New England Kitchen Magazine*, a visitor to a Georgia exposition described with a tingle of horrified relish the typical dinner she was served by a cordial Southern hostess: "Turnips cooked with pork, *green tops and all*, beef roasted to a cinder, and coffee of Chattahoochian flavor. . . ." Virtually the only food she could swallow during her stay was served at a reception in the Woman's Building of the exposition, where a domestic scientist from Boston was in charge of the menu. Bouillon in cups, "tiny crackers," plates of chicken salad with olives and a single roll, and a green-and-white gelatin dessert made up the familiar meal welcomed by this grateful traveler.

Many of the influential scientific cooks had been trained in Boston, or converted to domestic science by the example of a Boston cooking teacher, and their values were solidly based in New England cookery. New Englanders, as Professor Atwater liked to point out, had the instinctive good sense to "supplement the fat of their pork with the protein of beans and the carbohydrates of potatoes, and supplement maize and wheat flour with the protein of codfish and mackerel; and while subsisting largely on such frugal but rational diets, are well nourished, physically strong, and distinguished for their intellectual and moral force." The Scots, too, exhibited an admirable wisdom by eating quantities of oatmeal with their haddock and herring, Professor Atwater noted, but the poorer classes of India, China, parts of Italy and Germany, and much of the American South sustained themselves on too much carbohydrate with too little protein for adequate nourishment. These people, he concluded, "suffer physically, intellectually, and morally thereby." The scientific cooks who fanned across the country with their cookbooks and charts and lecture notes also carried with them highly specific dietary regimens for the citizens they observed and taught, and heading those regimens very often were the foods they associated with breakfast and dinner in New England. "To introduce soups and stews . . . roast beef, rare steak, Boston baked beans, Boston brown bread, codfish balls, creamed codfish, Johnny cake, Graham gems and hash was not by any means an easy task," admitted the teacher in charge of the domestic department at Atlanta University, after two years of supervising the diet of 130 black women students. Most of them had been raised in rural areas on "fat pork, hoe cake, pone, hominy and molasses," she explained, and they rejected with special abhorrence the soup and the baked beans. After the first year, however, the women began to grow more accustomed to the diet, and the teacher noticed an improvement in their health as well. "I can only urge patience upon anyone who undertakes to improve the dietary of any class of people," she advised her colleagues. "Allow at least two years for the seed most carefully sown and *covered* to come into sight, and keep up courage by remembering that *good* seed will surely sprout if you have properly prepared the ground." Ellen Richards, who kept an eye on the Atlanta dietary experiment, visited the university herself and was encouraged by the progress shown in the second year. "I went over the dietary very carefully," she reported later, "and it seems to be the greatest triumph we have had over unreasoning habit and natural distaste."

Another project in Northern cookery for Southern blacks took place in Norfolk, Virginia, where a New York cooking teacher taught up to forty-five girls a day and instructed their mothers in sewing as well. The founders of the school, three ladies who obtained the funds from a Northern philanthropist, were given the use of two rooms in a Norfolk public school, "and we immediately proceeded to elevate them with soap, sapolio and kalsomine," wrote one. They hung curtains, installed an organ, and required each young cook to wear a dark blue calico frock, a white apron, and a white cap.

> Thus we ensured cleanliness, the self respect that accompanies it, and the discipline which a uniform carries with it . . . [explained the founder]. The scholars marched to their places to the music of an organ. . . . We used the best cooking utensils. We taught them the best way of preparing food, even to garnishing the dishes with parsley, lemon, etc. . . . One day I was watching the work, and also the large group of spectators who came daily to visit the school, when one of the women stepped out of the crowd and whispered to me, "Oh, this is beautiful; I suppose this is what you call culture." Then I knew I had won my cause.

Teaching cookery according to New England standards was even harder for those domestic scientists who worked on Indian reservations than it was in the South, owing to the language problem and the constant shortage of supplies in remote areas. Nonetheless, the teachers who chose this work were proud of what they were able to accomplish. Their mission, as one expressed it, was to acquaint the Indian woman with the "refinements of a cultured home" and to help her experience "civilization and a taste of cleanly comfort." A teacher trained in Boston wrote to *New England Kitchen Magazine* from the "Arickaree" reservation in North Dakota to describe her success in teaching the women to bake bread—"crisp, brown loaves that would do credit to a Boston cooking school"—despite the fact that there had been no loaf pans, so that the bread had to be baked in tin cans. These "pretty round loaves," she added, were a perfect way to obtain "dainty circular slices for our poached eggs." More adventurous than some of her colleagues, she sent along "Mrs. Mary Bear's recipe" for squash baked with drippings and sugar, which she said tasted like nuts, or caramels, or "something good, I don't know just what." Local styles of cooking, however, were not normally praised when domestic science was taught to Indian girls. The syllabus distributed by the federal Office of Indian Affairs for teaching cookery in Indian schools was much like the outline for any public-school cookery course, with the customary emphasis on careful measuring, economical soups and croquettes, the importance of fruit at breakfast, and the "use and abuse" of desserts. Occasionally the syllabus recommended that the teacher invite a discussion of traditional customs, but only in order to highlight the differences between Indian and modern ways. In the lesson on bread, for example, the teacher was advised to start by asking the children to describe how bread was made in their own homes. "The primitive manner of grinding grain between stones, mixing the flour with water and baking on hot stones or before the fire will form a practical beginning," it was noted in the syllabus, "and will lead up to the flour of commerce which is purchased at the mills or stores and from which our bread is made."

One of the most impassioned and carefully nurtured of these efforts to regulate American eating habits was the New England Kitchen, a project that represented the best hopes of several leading domestic scientists and their philanthropic allies. The New England Kitchen—it had no affiliation with the magazine, but the magazine borrowed its name as a mark of affection—was the brainchild of Ellen Richards, whose dream was to woo the poor and working people of Boston away from their tawdry diets by selling them sanitary and economical food all cooked and ready to eat. What she had in mind was a friendly but strictly educational establishment where neighborhood people could purchase at low cost a few different soups and stews, perhaps a rice pudding or a nourishing broth for an invalid, and take the food home. All the cooking would be done in the open where customers could see it, under conditions of absolute cleanliness, and the food would be prepared with the best ingredients, plain though they might be. The most exciting part of the scheme for Mrs. Richards was the hope that the kitchen would provide, not only impeccable New England cookery, but absolutely invariable New England cookery. She wanted every portion of tomato soup and beef stew to be exactly the same from day to day, in terms of taste, texture, and nutritional value. The kitchen, as she saw it, ought to be an experiment station, very much like the agricultural experiment stations in which scientists carried on studies in animal feeding. Studies in human feeding were long overdue, Mrs. Richards believed, and she envisioned a cooking laboratory where rigorous experimentation would lead domestic scientists to the discovery of infallible methods for preparing the most inexpensive and nutritious dishes. Then, if these principles of exact cookery could be disseminated among the people, along with a taste of the food itself, the standardization of American eating habits might at last become possible.

Ellen Richards knew very well that scientific research of this sort, in which no certain results or successes could be assured on a timetable, would not attract philanthropic support as easily as those simpler charities that involved feeding the poor. She was pleased, therefore, to be backed up by two prominent Bostonians who sustained the work morally and financially and with unflagging faith. Her chief financial benefactor was Pauline Agassiz Shaw, one of the most generous and imaginative of the city's wealthy women reformers, who had spurred many projects in education for women and children. Mrs. Shaw gave Ellen Richards an essentially unrestricted grant to pursue studies in the "food and nutrition of workingmen and its possible relation to the question of the use of intoxicating liquors." This included subsidies for the purchase of laboratory apparatus as well, for which Mrs. Richards often expressed special appreciation. She had spent much of her own career helping women gain access to chemistry laboratories and scientific training, always against the general disapproval of the chemistry profession and the public; to have the best equipment now made available without question was an extra tribute she acknowledged with gratitude.

The other benefactor, whose presence was felt more strongly in the day-to-day activity of the kitchen, was Edward Atkinson, a Boston businessman, financier, and freelance expert on most of the important political and economic issues of his time. Late in his career, when he decided to turn his deliberate and inventive attentions to the problem of food, he had many more influential friends and acquaintances than most domestic scientists could claim, and was able to attract a great deal of respectful interest in his theories. After his retirement from business, Atkinson had the leisure and the financial means to pursue his ideas zealously, and he kept up an especially relentless campaign in favor of what he considered his breakthrough analysis of American eating problems. One day he had noticed a workman opening his dinner pail and taking out "a mess of cold victuals . . . which seems to me must require the digestive power of an ostrich to dispose of," he wrote in his 1896 text, *The Science of Nutrition*. A portable stove the size of a dinner pail, in which a workman could leave his food to cook by itself all morning, seemed to Atkinson a good solution; and he set about trying to make one. He had only partial success with this effort, but in the process he did invent something he believed would put the best and most easily prepared meals on every American table, if women could be persuaded to try it. This device he called the Aladdin Oven ("At the extraordinary manner in which the sumptuous repast was obtained the Princess could not conceal her astonishment.—Aladdin and the Wonderful Lamp"). An insulated box with moveable shelves, built to fit over a kerosene lamp, the Aladdin Oven operated for the most part on the principle of long, slow cooking. Oatmeals, soups, stews, cheap cuts of meat, root vegetables, and puddings could all be prepared this way, and the fuel cost was very little even when large quantities of food filled the oven. Describing his invention to the American Association for the Advancement of Science, Atkinson explained that when cooks used ordinary cast-iron stoves they were not able to regulate the heat and instead were forced to deal with the food itself. Watching, stirring, shifting the pans about, "and various other empirical devices" were the only ways to control the application of heat to the food. With the Aladdin Oven, however, even "persons of very moderate intelligence" could apply the right measure of heat to ensure thorough cooking and never touch the food. Atkinson also figured out ways to brown and broil and sauté using the oven, and claimed that everything from omelets to popovers received their best treatment in his device. (Deep-fat frying, he admitted, was probably not a good idea.) The advantages he cited were many: the oven was inexpensive to operate, didn't heat up the kitchen, cooked virtually anything with little work beforehand and no attention necessary during the cooking itself, allowed the natural flavors of food to develop so that sauces and spices were redundant, and produced far more sanitary meals than those handled constantly by a cook and subjected to all kinds of kitchen germs. The last point was an especially important one. Atkinson disliked seeing his cook make bread the traditional way, kneading it by hand—"I do not fancy paws and perspiration in my bread; the idea is unpleasant even to speak of"—and he introduced into his own kitchen a mechanical bread kneader, a mechanical bread raiser, and of course the oven. "Here are examples of bread which no human hand has touched even from the time the wheat was planted until it was taken from the pan in which the loaf was baked," he concluded triumphantly.

Ellen Richards was an early partisan of the Aladdin Oven, and she, too, delighted in the "cleanliness and daintiness" that it made possible in the kitchen. Handling food, she emphasized in a letter to Atkinson, was "distasteful to women," and added parenthetically, "Do you not believe that the extreme use of meat is at the bottom of this trouble— It can not be handled without disgust." When she set about organizing the New England Kitchen, Atkinson helped direct financial support her way, and the Aladdin Oven was in prominent use from the start. One of the first undertakings at the kitchen, in fact, was a series of experiments featuring the Aladdin Oven in the making of beef broth and pea soup. Under the direction of Mrs. Richards, domestic scientists at the kitchen tried several methods using different equipment—two other versions of an enclosed, slow-cooking oven were then on the market along with the Aladdin Oven—and found that the Aladdin Oven answered their needs perfectly. "We believe this to be the first time that standard dishes have ever been prepared on scientific principles with such exactness that they may be duplicated, in every particular, like an apothecary's prescription," Mrs. Richards reported after six months of experimentation. The Aladdin Oven was not completely ready to replace the usual cookstove, she conceded, but it was superior in many ways to any other apparatus in its ability to produce good, digestible food with simplicity and economy. Most American kitchens were dependent upon "crude and unreliable" stoves, she stressed, and it was impossible to achieve predictable results with such equipment.

Mrs. Richards's closest partner in the New England Kitchen was Mary Hinman Abel, a self-taught domestic scientist who studied, lectured, and wrote widely in the field. Artists were few in domestic science, but she was the movement's chief poet. One of her compositions, "Good Food for Little Money," was written at the time of the Chicago World's Fair and distributed there:

Good Food for Little Money

Oats, peas, beans, and barley grow,
Wheat and corn and rice for you,
Meat that's cheap, and eggs when low;
Milk with cream, without it too;
Wholesome cabbage, and greens, a few
To cook in the pot with the simmering stew;
And Erin's tuber, in seasons good,
When the price is low for this starchy food.

These are the things that first we buy
When the purse is low but courage high.
We do our work with muscles firm,
And bide the day till the tide shall turn,
But chops and roasts are not for us,
Nor eggs in winter; nor fruit the first
Of the seasons' gift; and small our share
Of that which rewards the gardener's care.

Mrs. Abel, who was married to a professor of pharmacology, had spent five years in Germany with her husband and had observed the European "people's kitchens," where for a few pennies anyone in the neighborhood could buy bread and soup or other simple preparations. She also acquainted herself with some of the nutritional research that was going on in Europe at the time, and made a special study of the thrifty ways practiced by German housekeepers. Back in the United States she assembled what she had learned abroad, along with the latest work done by Atwater, and entered an essay contest sponsored by the American Public Health Association on the topic of "practical sanitary and economic cooking adapted to persons of moderate and small means." The philanthropist Henry Lomb, of Bausch and Lomb, was offering a $500 first prize and a $200 second prize. There were seventy submissions but Mrs. Abel's won handily—none of the others even came close enough to merit the second prize—and the Lomb Prize Essay, as it was called, was published by the American Public Health Association in book form. "Even a casual reader of that title-page cannot fail to see to what an unnumbered host it would appeal," wrote Isabel Bevier in her history of the home-economics movement. " 'Practical!' 'economic,' 'moderate means'—what words to conjure with as regards the universal demand for food!"

The Lomb Prize Essay was a concisely written account of the basics of scientific cookery, including recipes and menu suggestions. Mrs. Abel also drew on her knowledge of Europe to offer special instructions for feeding a family on the remarkably small sum of thirteen cents a day per person. "All observing travelers unanimously give this as much of his large wage as the foreigner does of his small testimony,—'If our American workman knew how to make one, he could live in luxury,' " she wrote, and queried rhetorically, "But what are the special lessons to be learned of the foreign housewife? We answer, chiefly self-denial and saving." The thirteen-cent menus she offered in this spirit consisted very largely of carbohydrates, especially bread, as in one day's ration of "flour pancakes" (pancakes made without eggs) for breakfast; bread soup, noodles, stew, and rice pudding for dinner; and flour soup, fried bread, cheese, and toast for supper. "I only ask you in advance to try the recipes I shall give and to try to lay aside your prejudices against dishes to which you are not accustomed, as soups and cheese dishes for instance," she begged her readers. "You cannot afford to reject anything that will vary your diet, for many good tasting things you cannot buy."

One of the judges for the Lomb Prize Essay contest was Ellen Richards, who did not know Mrs. Abel but shared her point of view on just about every issue raised in the essay. She was so impressed by the prize-winning essay that as soon as she made the writer's acquaintance she urged her to come to Boston to help start the New England Kitchen. Mrs. Abel was living in Michigan at the time, but she agreed to leave home for six months and work with Mrs. Richards. Very quickly the two women became partners and good friends. A shop on the corner of Pleasant and Winchester Streets in downtown Boston was rented and outfitted, and on January 24, 1890, the kitchen opened for business. The menu was small at first, for Mrs. Richards would not permit anything to be sold until Mrs. Abel, working with an assistant, had experimented long enough to come up with the most nutritious, inexpensive, and efficient recipe possible. Beef broth (18 cents a quart), beef stew (12 cents), three kinds of soup (12 cents), oatmeal or corn mush (5 cents), and Indian pudding (15 cents) were among the first dishes available; and although it was possible at the time to buy a full meal, of sorts, for as little as ten cents at a restaurant, these prices were certainly fair for the indisputable food value. Nothing was added to the menu until Mrs. Richards was convinced that it could be offered in good faith as the best and the cheapest.

Atkinson, who was eager for the kitchen to begin baking his favorite sterile bread in the Aladdin Ovens, kept after Mrs. Richards to try his recipes, but she felt it was wiser to wait. Bread was crucial to the success of an economical eating plan, but Americans showed such a definite preference for white, puffy bread that Mrs. Richards hesitated to try to impose healthier loaves until the other foods from the kitchen had been tasted and appreciated. "Certainly we are now nearly ready to attack the bread question," she wrote to him three months after the opening. "I had not forgotten it but I wished to get the thorough good will of every body without arousing any opposition before we touched such a sore point. We see we must win ardent believers in us in order to get our wares fairly tested. . . . Mrs. Abel is winning the confidence of the people. . . ." Three months later the impatient Atkinson baked a few loaves himself and sent them to Mrs. Richards. They were wholesome, sweet, and rich, she assured him, but just a bit too heavy to be absolutely acceptable. His bread weighed fully a pound more than loaves of the same size sold in bakeries, she pointed out, and people did like their bread to be light. By the end of the year, however, white bread and "health bread" had been perfected and added to the kitchen's menu.

According to an appreciative article in *The Century*, written by Maria Parloa, the people of Boston took to the kitchen gladly.

> Between eleven and one o'clock men, women, and children of all sorts and conditions come and go [she wrote]. A well-dressed gentleman takes a quart jar from his handbag, and has it filled. Is it for himself, or is he a doctor who is taking this nutritious and savory beef-broth to a patient? A feeble old man brings in his pail to be filled. Dainty-looking young women, who perhaps are workers in shops, or teachers, or possibly students who provide their own meals, take away in their shopping-bags soups, stews, chowders, pressed beef, and health bread. Little children, black and white come with their pails, plates, bowls, and pitchers. Old and middle-aged women appear, some apparently prosperous, and others with the stamp of poverty and hard work fixed upon them. . . . The perfect cleanliness, the gracious manner in which customers are served, the quiet, order, neatness, and despatch with which the vast amount of work is done, are marvelous.

This and similarly gratifying publicity drew the attention of reformers and philanthropists all over the country, and the progress of the kitchen was watched with great interest. Jane Addams sent a settlement worker from Chicago to study the operation of the kitchen and confer with Mrs. Richards, and then set up a similar establishment at Hull-House. Another group opened a kitchen in Providence, the philanthropist T. A. Havemeyer was persuaded to support one in New York City, and in Rochester the Women's Educational and Industrial Union began to investigate the possibility of opening one. By the end of the second year a branch of the original kitchen had been set up in Boston's North End, cooking classes for neighborhood women and for medical students were under way at the Pleasant Street headquarters, and the kitchen was sending out insulated hot lunches to shopgirls, teachers, and factory workers upon request.

The high point of its fame was reached when Mrs. Richards was invited to create a New England Kitchen as part of the Massachusetts state exhibit at the Chicago World's Fair. A small clapboard house was erected on the exposition grounds near the anthropology exhibit—"a fitting place," remarked *New England Kitchen Magazine*, "since the development of the human race is largely dependent upon food." Inside, she set up a scientific kitchen outfitted with an Aladdin Oven and some of the other equipment used in the New England Kitchen, a small library of domestic-science literature, a few tables where light, balanced lunches were served, and a counter where samples of the food could be purchased to take home. The walls were lined with menus, charts, and diagrams; an array of leaflets on scientific cookery was available; and inspirational mottoes ("Wherefore do you spend money for that which is not bread, and your labor for that which satisfieth not?") were framed and hung all over the house.

For Mrs. Richards one of the most satisfying aspects of the exhibit, along with the opportunity to introduce the principles of scientific cookery to the public on a grand scale, was the chance it gave her to honor one of her personal saints and a hero of the domestic-science movement: Count Rumford. "I propose to make this quite in the nature of a Centennial celebration of his work," she told Atkinson, "which impresses me more and more as I read it over now." Count Rumford was an American—he was born Benjamin Thompson in 1753—who lived in New England studying science and doing experiments on his own until he was forced to leave the country "owing to certain political complications," as Mrs. Richards put it in an essay she wrote about him. In truth, he was probably a spy for the British during the Revolution, and he served in the British Army after his banishment from the colonies. Later he took a position in the retinue of Karl Theodor, ruler of Bavaria—"the King of England having graciously given his permission," Mrs. Richards wrote. Again, he was most likely sent to Bavaria to be a spy, but his assignment gave him the opportunity to apply some of his scientific theories on a practical basis. Karl Theodor set him to improving the morale and discipline of the army, and to that end Thompson developed insulated clothing, put the army to work on public projects, housed the men with their families, provided education, music, and sports, and introduced the potato into their diet. During this period he invented the kitchen range—essentially enclosing the fireplace and chimney in an insulated box—and designed more efficient pots and pans. His next assignment was to free Bavaria from its large population of beggars, and he did this by introducing organized charity. On January 1, 1790—a day when beggars were out in force because it was the traditional day for almsgiving—the military arrested every beggar in Munich and had each one fill out a questionnaire. Then they were told to return the next day and report to a huge workhouse where they would be given employment, food, and cash grants when necessary. Most of the city's 2,600 beggars came regularly to the workhouse, an establishment that included schools, living quarters, and a dining hall outfitted with Rumford's stove and utensils. The beggars produced army uniforms as their chief occupation, and after a few years of sponsoring this experiment, the national treasury showed a profit of six pounds per beggar per year. For his achievement Benjamin Thompson was made Count Rumford.

Returning to England he established the Royal Institution for scientific research, and continued his writing and experimenting. He developed the notion of measuring fuel energy in terms of heat, although he didn't call his unit the calorie; he worked to improve his stove by making it continually more fuel-efficient; he created the drip coffeepot, the double boiler, and the tea kettle; and he tried diligently to popularize the use of corn in England. Married briefly to Madame Lavoisier, he moved to France toward the end of his life and died there in 1814. Count Rumford was apparently a crotchety and unpleasant person, and despite the fact that his achievements were widely recognized and appreciated, he was not missed. According to his eulogy, "It was without loving or esteeming his fellow creatures that he had done them all these services."

Mrs. Richards and many other domestic scientists remembered Count Rumford most gratefully as the man who married science to practicality, applying the full force of his intellect to problems of cooking, eating, and domestic life. In their minds he was the real progenitor of the New England Kitchen, for one of his innovations at the Bavarian beggars' workhouse was a staple food that came to be called Rumford Soup. For a penny a day every Bavarian beggar could be fed on a pound and a half of soup made with peas, barley, and bread, and could be given an extra seven ounces of bread to take home. Mrs. Richards calculated that the soup as Rumford prepared it would have provided about 540 calories per pound, hardly a substantial ration, but enough, she wrote, "to afford a subsistence to the not very ambitious vagrants." Striving as she was to achieve a similar soup based on modern chemistry, Mrs. Richards had hoped to call the first kitchen on Pleasant Street the "Rumford Food Laboratory." She was dissuaded, according to one history of the kitchen, when others convinced her that such a name would "puzzle and repel" the people she was trying to reach. But she had no such constraints when she began to plan the World's Fair exhibit, and she proudly called it the Rumford Kitchen. Her chemical analysis of Rumford Soup was displayed on a chart there, Rumford's books were available in the library, and Mrs. Richards's own biographical essay about him was printed up in a leaflet and distributed.

After the World's Fair, and after the excitement of the Rumford Kitchen had died down, the fortunes of the New England Kitchen and its several imitators plummeted. The original kitchen was able to survive by obtaining contracts to provide lunches regularly to several institutions, including MIT and some of the public schools. But its branch in the North End, as well as the kitchens in Providence and New York, were failures—people simply did not buy the food. "It was disheartening when our favorite dishes, wholesome, nutritious and cheap, stayed unsold on the counter, though freshly prepared day after day, and when our most scientific receipts produced food that was uneatable . . ." admitted Mrs. Richards three years after the opening of the first kitchen. In a report written that same year for Pauline Agassiz Shaw, their benefactor, Mrs. Abel analyzed some of the factors that led to these disappointing results. "Those who come, do so regularly, but the number of those who are intelligent enough to appreciate the nature of the food is too few," she wrote of the North End branch. In Providence the kitchen had been set up in a manufacturing area inhabited by French and Irish immigrants, "the most incorrigible of all the communities," as Mrs. Abel described them. "One good-natured, affectionate Irish mother, when pressed to take an Indian pudding home to her children, replied, 'My boy says, "Oh! you can't make a Yankee of me that way!"' Here is the difficulty in a nutshell. . . ." Mrs. Abel was beginning to fear that it was not possible to arrive at a standard dish that would appeal to such "mixed nationalities and varied tastes" as were found in American cities. Moreover, even native-born citizens showed little interest in the pea soups and custards prepared at the kitchens.

> We began to ask, What are the national dishes of Americans? It is astonishing how few still partake of the simple fare known as New England. It seems to be a part of the restless and hurried life of this generation in large cities to have abandoned the cheap and simple foods that need long cooking and a little skill to make them palatable. This reduces the fare to chops and steaks, and tea with bread and cakes to be picked up at the bake-shop. Are these our national foods? It would almost seem so.

Neither Mrs. Abel nor Mrs. Richards was willing to give up her belief in the food they had so laboriously perfected, but both agreed that they had to change targets. The poor, the ignorant, and the working classes obviously were not ready for the New England Kitchen: they didn't appreciate the extraordinary sanitary conditions that the women insisted on maintaining in every kitchen, and they didn't care about the nutritional balance of the food. "The person who said, 'I don't want to eat what's good for me, I'd rather eat what I'd rather,' represents a large class," Mrs. Abel conceded. If American eating habits were going to change, the women decided, that change would have to begin at another level of society. The original New England Kitchen was still managing to sell small quantities of food to office employees, saleswomen, and "brain-workers" in downtown Boston, and it was supplying lunches very successfully to nine of the city's public high schools. These more educated workers on the fringe of the middle class, as well as the young people whose habits were not yet formed, seemed to constitute the most flexible group. Edward Atkinson, too, became convinced that the poor could not be helped at such an early stage of dietary reform. "The taste of the very poor whom it is most desirable to aid in economy of food, has become so depraved and they are so prejudiced in favor of the finest flour and the high priced meats, as to make it a useless undertaking to try to reach *them* . . ." he wrote to T. A. Havemeyer, the benefactor of the New York Kitchen. Good, nourishing food at low prices should be made available to "shop girls, the lower grade of teachers, decorators, young men just starting in life who possess intelligence but who earn very little money, etc., etc. . . ." he advised the philanthropist. "In that we have made steady progress and those to whom I first referred will ultimately be reached by a sifting down of information and by example. These jealous and suspicious working people in the lower grade will imitate their neighbors . . . while they utterly reject instruction such as we have undertaken to give them as one may say from above." The New York Kitchen, however, did not survive long enough to amass the kind of clientele Atkinson had in mind, much less to allow any dietary information to trickle down to the neighbors.

Scientific cookery itself had not been discredited by the failure of the kitchens; on the contrary, the excellent publicity generated by the New England Kitchen and the

Rumford Kitchen, along with the support of admired men like Edward Atkinson and Professor Atwater, helped to create a new and impressive public respect for dietary matters. Domestic scientists were being sought not only as teachers but as experts, and in the field of institutional feeding their participation became especially prominent. Many were invited to examine the diets of hospital patients, prisoners, asylum inmates, college students, and other groups subjected to quantity cooking on a small budget, and to make recommendations for improving the nutritional quality of the food at the lowest cost. After their disillusioning experience with the mass of poor and working people, Mrs. Richards and her colleagues welcomed the opportunity to work with these more captive populations.

The sick, in particular, seemed as though they should be amenable to change, since proper diet would, in fact, hasten their recovery and thus prompt their trust in foods they might never try if they were healthy. "No better school of diet could be found than an intelligently managed hospital," Mrs. Richards declared. Patients accustomed to corned beef and cabbage might be introduced very effectively to chicken soup, she maintained, at least if it could be served on the wards with an "atmosphere of good cheer and confidence" provided by the nurses. (She did, however, acknowledge a new respect for the use of familiar flavors in preparing food that people would have to be induced to eat. The absence of garlic and salt pork in many recipes had helped to doom the New England Kitchen.) Her emphasis on the crucial importance of diet in caring for the sick, which had always been a major focus of the domestic-science movement, came as a novelty to many hospitals, which were paying only slightly less attention to their patients' food than hospitals do today. One study of Italian immigrants in Chicago found that many of them stayed away from hospitals entirely, because they were so averse to the food, and that those who had to remain long on a hospital ward were unable to eat anything and complained of constant hunger. The report recommended that a "few harmless concessions" to their native taste in food be granted at the beginning of the stay in order to make such patients more willing and tractable. After a few days they might look more favorably upon broth and milk toast, and gradually put their bad habits behind them. "Perhaps the treatment of an Italian during this period of change should be studied much as the treatment of an inebriate being won from his strong drink is studied," suggested the investigator.

The recuperative powers of a scientific diet were often imagined to be moral as well as physical, a hope that more than justified the hiring of domestic scientists to scrutinize the food served in prisons, reformatories, workhouses, and asylums. "The increased interest in the study of foods and their effects has led philanthropists to look upon a wholesome diet as a possible agent in the reformation of criminals," observed *New England Kitchen Magazine*. "Suitable food in early life doubtless would make respectable citizens of many boys and girls who otherwise become charges of the city or state." At the request of the mayor of Boston, Mrs. Richards undertook an investigation of nine city institutions and came up with several recommendations for new dietary standards for the inmates. Prisoners, she instructed, who were likely to be able-bodied but sedentary, should be kept away from "stimulating" foods: they were best fed on a bland diet of bread and vegetables, with very little meat, and the use of spices and condiments should be sharply restricted. "While the food should be well cooked, so that it may be palatable and easily digested, it is not wise to make the menu so attractive as to encourage petty crimes for the sake of good fare," she warned. Able-bodied adults living in almshouses should receive the same nourishing but deliberately unappealing diet as prisoners, she advised, while old people or the infirm—"who come to it in many cases from no fault of their own"—should be provided with more milk and sugar, along with dried fruits and an occasional egg. Children, sick people, and the insane deserved the most generous rations, in her estimation, although in no case did she advise spending more than eleven cents a day per person. It was usually figured by domestic scientists at that time that a man doing moderate work could be fed adequately for about twenty cents a day or less, if his wife knew how to buy and cook economically, so Mrs. Richards's recommendations were strict even with the benefit of wholesale purchasing taken into consideration. Under conditions of such rigid economy, she pointed out, it was possible that inmates with "personal idiosyncrasies" about food might actually starve, especially in the children's institutions. She urged medical inspectors to watch out for such cases.

Of all the dietary-reform measures undertaken in this era, the most aggressively rational was a series of nationwide investigations sponsored by the federal government and carried out very often by hand-picked teams of domestic scientists. Since 1886 Professor Atwater and other researchers had been collecting information about American eating habits directly from a sample of dinner tables in New England, Philadelphia, and Chicago. This early research was on a very limited scale, but in 1894 the Department of Agriculture agreed to fund the work on a more comprehensive and systematic basis. Under the direction of Professor Atwater, domestic scientists began moving into the kitchens of families across the country to find out exactly what people were eating and how their diets could be improved. These investigations were as objective as the researchers could make them—they entered every home as if it were a laboratory and the family a set of caged mice—but the mission was no less inspiring for its scientific rigor. Their dream with this new work was to guide all families toward Atwater's nutritional standard for Americans: between 90 and 150 grams of protein per day, and up to 4,500 calories, depending on the amount of physical labor performed.

The earliest dietary investigations had concentrated chiefly upon poor people, laborers, factory workers, and others living on the smallest incomes. With the onset of federal funding, however, Atwater increased the scope of the studies to include people of every class, not only because the basic research would be of value, but because most reformers believed that poor nutrition and wasteful buying and cooking were just as prevalent in the business and professional classes as among laborers and slum dwellers. Eventually over five hundred studies were done, in twenty-two states and territories. The groups that were scrutinized by Atwater's field workers included college students and rural families in Georgia; lumbermen in Maine; infants, athletes, and "fruitarians" in California; farmers in Vermont; Bible students in Massachusetts; blacks in Virginia; and hill families in Tennessee. After collecting the information, the investigators would write up their findings for bulletins that were published by the Department of Agriculture and distributed throughout the country to teachers, magazine food editors, women's clubs, charity and reform workers, and others with an interest in what Atwater termed the "pecuniary economy of food."

In a typical dietary study the investigator—usually a domestic-science teacher, or a young woman with a degree in chemistry—first had to persuade the family to participate. In this she was often assisted by a local settlement house; it was also helpful to offer a small sum of money. Once the family had agreed, the investigator began her work by weighing every item of food they possessed. "Eternal vigilance is the price of knowledge in dietary studies," stressed Isabel Bevier, who undertook several of them as a chemistry student of Atwater's. In a speech about her work to a group of domestic scientists in Boston, she explained that precise records of every food item on hand or purchased in the course of the study were essential. At the end of the study all the food remaining in the house was weighed and the result subtracted from the original total; thus it was possible to determine the amount of food consumed during the study. While the investigator did not have to be present for every meal, she did have to visit frequently enough to weigh all the new purchases, and Miss Bevier noted that these were excellent opportunities for the scientist to gather data informally about the family's living habits.

The measurement of waste was equally important,

since the investigators hoped to impress upon each family the sizable amount of nutritious material that was thrown into the garbage during cooking, or left on the plates after the meal. The investigator who could not personally collect and weigh the garbage from each meal was supposed to instruct the wife very carefully on how to do it, or at least to ask her to set aside food remnants until they could be picked up. It seemed impractical even to the indefatigable Atwater for an investigator to attempt to collect the "solid excreta from the food," but he waited eagerly for the day when dietary studies would include records of digestion as well as consumption. At the end of the study, the investigator was able to figure exactly what the family had consumed in the form of protein, carbohydrate, and fat, and at how great an expense. With this data in hand she might then sit down with the wife for what Miss Bevier called a "frank talk" and offer some tactful advice.

The nature of this advice can be guessed from the published versions of the dietary investigations, which included not only the tables computing each family's nutritional intake but a brief discussion evaluating the diet and suggesting improvements. In one Pittsburgh family studied by Miss Bevier, a household of nine headed by a consumptive blacksmith, the diet centered on potatoes, bread, and cheap cuts of beef. Miss Bevier admitted that it would have been difficult to spend less on food than this family did—about nine cents a day per person—but she singled out a few possibilities for improvement. Among other food purchases, the family spent $3.45 in the course of the month on round steak, pork loin, a bit of bacon and boiled ham, a few oysters, and four pounds of cheese. If they had eliminated these items, much the liveliest in their diet, and purchased instead ten pounds of oatmeal, seventeen pounds of beans, ninety-four pounds of potatoes, forty-seven pounds of flour, and nine pounds of beef rump, they would have spent the same amount of money but increased their nutrients greatly. Miss Bevier thought that if "proper care" were applied to the cooking, the new diet would be just as appealing; but she gave no hint as to how ten pounds of oatmeal and ninety-four pounds of potatoes might be thus transformed without, for example, purchasing any milk or butter.

There were many logical and statistical shortcomings in Atwater's investigatory method, but perhaps its chief weakness was an insistent faith in method itself, which led investigators to ignore anything that could not be tabulated. In truth, it was impossible to assess the diets of women and children during these studies, because the method called for the entire intake of a family to be computed on the basis of nutrients consumed "per man per day." Once the investigator had figured the total amount of nutrients consumed by a family in a month, that is, she divided the total to find the quantities consumed per person per day. Then, since a woman was supposed to require only four-fifths of the food needed by a man, and children of different ages required proportionally less, the investigator assumed that these requirements were actually met. She reduced the family to a mythical "man" consuming all the month's nutrients over a longer span of time, taking it for granted that every family divided its food at the dinner table according to the official proportions recommended by scientists. What seems more likely, however, is that the man, or the chief wage-earners, would have been fed as adequately as possible and that the children and finally the wife would have eaten what was left. This method also discouraged the investigator from taking into account the extra nutritional needs of women during pregnancy or when breast-feeding. Atwater described the studies as involving families "normal" for their class and circumstances, but gave no indication as to whether pregnancy and lactation fell within those bounds.

Finally, the work done by women and children could not be charted in these studies—the tables left no room for such "atypical" facts—which meant that their real nutritional requirements could not be acknowledged. The dietary standards that Atwater set—which recommended a certain amount of protein and a certain number of calories per day according to the amount of work performed

—ranged from a low of 2,400 calories (for a woman at light muscular exercise) to a high of 4,500 calories (for a man at hard muscular work). The only designations for women's daily activity, however, were "light muscular exercise" and "moderate muscular work," and the nutritional requirements for the latter were exactly the same as those for a man seated at a desk. Similarly, children were assumed to be at leisure, no matter what their economic circumstances were. Studying the diets of black tenant farmers in Alabama, then, the investigators noted that women and children often worked in the fields alongside the men, but since there was no way according to the method to take that work into consideration, or to assign nutritional needs to it, they decided for convenience's sake to assume that it didn't exist. In another series of investigations, done in New York City, women who had the job of housekeeper in their tenements and cleaned the buildings for a reduction in rent were classed in terms of their nutritional needs with women who did only their own housework. The families in which women did this extra work sometimes showed a greater consumption of food than the investigator thought necessary, so generally the family was advised to eat less.

In the very blindness of their efficiency, these dietary investigations helped boost domestic scientists to a new height of self-respect. The clean and precise task of gathering information for scientific analysis could not possibly be confused with cooking, much less eating, and the institutional backing of the federal government gave the work an orderliness and a magnitude that surpassed their most ambitious reveries. To have acknowledged individual quirks like pregnancy or child labor would only have interrupted the smooth operation of the intellectual machinery, and dragged down the whole process into a slough of those idiosyncratic emotional responses traditionally called female. Committed as they were to a future bound on all sides by science, these reformers thought of themselves as missionaries for progress, leading their frightened sisters into the modern world and helping them cast aside the sentiments that tied them to old habits. And like missionaries, they worked most effectively by their own standards when they kept their eyes fixed upon a single narrow ray of truth. Some of the other reformers and writers of that era looked to the past for their inspiration, seeking to restore an elusive American golden age of simple values and country ways; but to domestic scientists the rural past was an ignominious failure and the golden age was ahead. The reformer Helen Campbell complained that women raised in villages and on farms—"from Maine to Oregon, wherever the American pioneer had settled"—delivered more children to the insane asylums than any other class of women and were themselves doomed to a living degeneracy. "Her teeth fall; her hair falls off; her skin grows leathery . . . Nine times out of ten she has never heard of salad, and is incapable of a soup, and her family subsist on fried meat, chiefly pork, and on pie and cake three times a day." This woman, the victim of what Mrs. Campbell called the "home kitchen and its absolutely destructive products," had nothing to gain from tradition. If domestic science could encourage her to transform that kitchen into a laboratory and to raise her children according to Atwater's standards, then the way to a glittering future would be opened. The "bruised and weary pilgrims" who made up the female population of America, in Mrs. Campbell's eyes, would find redeeming solace at last, not in some cloudy realm of angelic domesticity, but in Madison, Ann Arbor, or Palo Alto, where universities were planning their courses in household science.

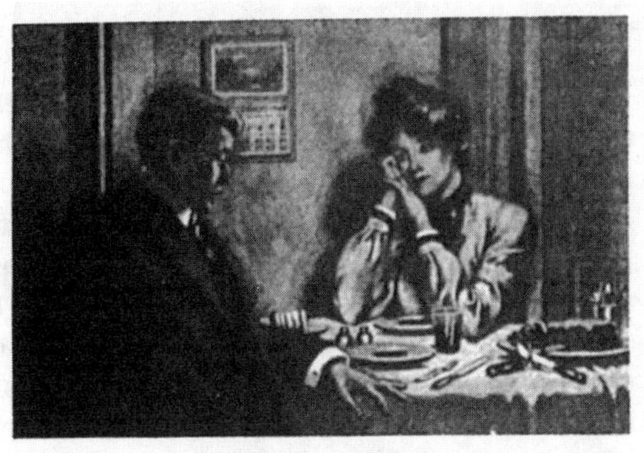

Seven
Foes in Our Own Household

During the first days of the twentieth century, Ellen Richards wrote down some of her dreams for the home, the kitchen, and the dinner of the future. In an article called "Housekeeping in the Twentieth Century" she conjured up a house assembled by mass production but nonetheless carefully suited to the individual family and expressive of the family's personality, where the domestic machinery ran smoothly and quietly. Tightly fitted walls kept out dust and vermin, and the factory-made furniture was cheap, leaving the family with more money for books and "intellectual pleasures." The real head of this house was the mistress—Mrs. Richards saw the master spending a lot of time at his club—who ran the house comfortably by herself, employing no servants. With the help of a telephone and a "household register" listing the names of all the service personnel she might need, the entire establishment was under her control. A "competent assistant" might be hired to help with the children if she could afford it; otherwise she devoted most of her own time to caring for them, knowing she could resume her other interests after ten years or so.

"Her children will not require so much care as ours are apt to exact," Mrs. Richards claimed; she was sure that the calm, sanitary surroundings in which they were raised would keep them as healthy and happy as animals. Every new scientific device that might save steps and labor was installed in the kitchen, the pantry held a large stock of prepared foods, and a pneumatic tube connected the kitchen with a supply station. If an emergency arose, or an unexpected guest arrived, there was no disruption of household routine: the supply station sent anything requested within ten minutes. All this convenience in the kitchen was possible only because food was produced in quantity by machine, just as furniture and clothing were produced, and Mrs. Richards was aware that the strongest objections to her vision of the future would be roused by the idea of "bread made by the yard, and pies by the hundred." People didn't mind buying tables and chairs that came from factories, but she knew they expected more "individuality" from their meals. "I grant that each family has a weakness for the flavor produced by its own kitchen bacteria," she acknowledged, "but that is a prejudice due to lack of education." In time, she was confident, people would grow to appreciate the superior cleanliness and consistency that only a factory kitchen staffed by skilled workers could provide.

At the time she set down these thoughts, Mrs. Richards was at last growing discouraged with the scattershot reform efforts aimed at one or another limited population. Just before writing this article she had visited the women's dining halls at the University of Chicago and returned home to Boston feeling unusually glum and pessimistic. The women at the university were being fed according to the best standard she knew, for not only was the Dean of Women firmly committed to domestic science but the central kitchen serving the women's dormitories had been outfitted with all the cooking equipment from the Rumford Kitchen after the close of the Chicago World's Fair. Nevertheless, she wrote to Edward

Atkinson, students were sending letters to the president of the university and to the Dean of Women demanding more "steak & chops & desserts," seemingly unable to accustom themselves to the boiled meats, tapioca puddings, and prunes that had been organized for them. "Much of the complaint is quite unfounded as we very well know, but it only shows how hopeless it all is until a better state of public opinion exists," she told Atkinson, and added with some frustration, "The world is wedded to its food which is killing off thousands who fondly believe that another cause is acting."

Mrs. Richards and some of her colleagues in the domestic-science movement were coming to believe that they had made two important errors in perception. First, as they learned from the New England Kitchen, the poor were not willing to be reformed and would only undergo their necessary moral redevelopment if the middle class showed the way. What Mrs. Richards called the "leaven of progress" now had to be applied, not to the slum dwellers or to the aristocracy, but to the "majority of the most intelligent American families"—the young professionals and their wives, who were starting up their homes on a salary of two to five thousand dollars a year. These middle-class families, she decided, constituted the "class to work for." Educated and alert, they already possessed the correct ideals and they understood the necessity for "sane and wholesome living." All they lacked was a certain amount of training and guidance to help them realize those ideas on a small budget.

To a great extent, of course, many of the lessons in right living generated by the domestic-science movement had been aimed at this very class of young people all along, especially in the realm of domestic-science fiction. "Tom and Sally," a popular twosome who starred in a serial that ran in *Good Housekeeping* in 1885, begin domestic life on Tom's modest salary as a bank clerk with the mutual agreement that if they cannot live economically in their own home, they will have to move to a boardinghouse. Boarding was a very common solution to the problem of finding an affordable home that could be managed without the cost of servants—so common that some domestic reformers, including Mrs. Richards, feared the boardinghouse eventually would replace the private home. Sally is determined to prove that she can make a better home than a boardinghouse can provide, and at less expense; and because she has been taught the principles of economy and nutrition she succeeds with gratifying swiftness. Her main weapon is her cooking: she makes plain, easily digested meals that Tom at first dislikes, brought up as he has been on pies and doughnuts. " 'I can make delightful pies, better than any you ever ate, but it's against my principles to make them,' " Sally explains. Tom quickly finds that he works much better at the bank upon this simple diet, which leaves him so clear-headed even after dinner that he is able to take on extra work to do at night. Financial savings and professional advancement follow soon after.

This theme, long in the emotional background of the domestic-science movement, finally emerged as an explicit definition of the movement's social goals. With it came a new and highly critical look at the role of Sally, for the second error of the early years had been a mistaken assumption about American women. As they traveled and taught and lectured across the country, the leading domestic scientists were becoming convinced that it was the woman of the family who had to be blamed for holding back the progress of the whole household. They had taken for granted that once the average wife was taught to think scientifically about cooking and cleaning, a new convert would have been won and another family saved from sickness and degradation. But women seemed to be balking. It was true that food and housekeeping magazines, cooking courses, and domestic-science school programs enjoyed great success, but as the experts could tell from their travels, there were still thousands of wives who remained untouched or who were picking up only the most superficial notions of progressive domesticity. Helen Campbell told the story, all too familiar to domestic scientists on the lecture circuit, of the scientific-cooking expert who was asked what her audiences throughout the country most frequently wanted to hear more about, after the lecture was over. "Chocolate cake and lemon pie," was the grim response. In the experience of these reformers, American women were still clinging to their grandmothers' and mothers' ways of housekeeping: they refused to understand the new appliances, insisted on serving heavy desserts, and threw out their leftovers instead of making soups. Much to Edward Atkinson's particular annoyance, moreover, they could not be persuaded to buy the Aladdin Oven, even though he had designed it especially to save them time, money, and labor. The prospect of making a virtually unlimited amount of pea soup at low cost was not arousing the response he had predicted. Like all reformers, the domestic scientists had to confront the irritatingly slow pace of real change, which seemed all the more frustrating in view of the large audiences they commanded and the favorable publicity that surrounded their work.

The failure of the National Household Economic Association was a special blow, for it had been founded in the excitement and optimism of the Chicago World's Fair as the organization that would mobilize the nation's thousands of clubwomen for domestic science. Women's clubs devoted to the study of history, foreign culture, and the arts had been thriving in towns and cities of every size for two decades at the time of the 1893 World's Fair, and the NHEA was supposed to work through these existing clubs, inducing their members to spend a year writing papers on household economics instead of on Shakespeare or horticulture or home life in Armenia. Despite constant prodding, however, club members rarely committed themselves to the study of housekeeping wholeheartedly enough to satisfy the NHEA. In 1902 the massive bienniale convention of the General Federation of Women's Clubs managed to produce only one paper on domestic science, and shortly afterward the NHEA gracefully turned over its work to a standing committee of the federation and disappeared. Trying to analyze why the NHEA never attracted much of an active membership, Anna Barrows of *New England Kitchen Magazine* argued that most women did feel sympathetic to the general cause of reforming the household but had no desire to change their own ways. "It is usually much easier to reform heathen at a distance than those at our own doors," Miss Barrows told an annual meeting of the flagging NHEA. She titled her speech "Foes in Our Own Household" and made it clear that the worst enemies in the modern home were the innate conservatism and inertia of women themselves. Women, she stressed, were not accustomed to thinking for themselves and had not been educated to understand the value of new ideas. "The devotion to family recipes for foods is amazing when we compare it with our custom regarding clothing," she noted. "Few of us would care to cut our garments by the patterns our grandmothers used." Most housekeepers were "servile imitators" of the past, who could neither organize nor plan but operated their homes according to whim and emergency. Without training in business, they had no understanding of money or of the value of their own time, and lacking the scientific spirit, they were practically superstitious in their adherence to tradition.

Helen Campbell was even more ferocious in attacking women for the sorry conditions of their own homes and families, and for refusing to admit progress into their lives. One by one the manufacturing industries that used to take place in the home and at woman's hand had slipped away, Mrs. Campbell pointed out in her text on household economics, and now they belonged in the provenance of men and technology. Only cooking and cleaning remained with women; consequently, these chores still existed in a state of "incoherent primitiveness." Meanwhile, "social problems of every order, born of this gross ignorance and indifference, press upon us and clamor for a solution the untrained mind can never give. . . ." She summed up the situation with a little aphorism that Ellen Richards thereafter quoted with great relish: "Man saw a better way, used and perfected it. Woman saw only the day's work." Ellen Richards was probably the most vehement of all the domestic scientists on this topic, and she harangued her own sex relentlessly. In her view women had to wake up, face new ideas, accept the help that science and technology offered, and give up the irrationality that characterized femininity. "Women have lacked respect for nature and her laws," she complained. "They have feared the thunder and ignored the microbe. They have the habit of shrieking at the sight of a toad and they get off a street car facing backward. Women cannot see why water will not run up hill. . . . They have allowed the sink drain to feed the well and the dark, damp cellar to furnish air to the house. . . . They need the influence of the scientific spirit, which tests all things and *suspends judgment*." On one occasion a friend wrote an apologetic letter to Mrs. Richards, explaining that while homemaking was "near my heart" and received a great deal of her time and strength, she and the others in her women's club preferred to study topics "as far as possible removed from housework" when they got together. All of them, she reported, were already good housekeepers, and they appreciated a chance to talk about history and poetry instead. Mrs. Richards marked out that section of the letter with firm strokes of her pen. "Are they?" she scribbled in the margin, next to the claim that the women were good housekeepers. "Must we not make them dissatisfied?" She was determined to criticize women until they knew enough to criticize themselves. Mrs. Richards became so well known for her impatience with her own sex that even a few of her colleagues urged her to tone down her rhetoric once in a while. "Make us seriously enthusiastic, intelligently hopeful, concretely helpful and kindly affectioned one toward another!" begged a woman to whom Mrs. Richards had sent an early draft of a speech. "Please do not say that she is not reliable and has no settled reverence for law," wrote another critic of the same speech. "Considering her opportunities, it seems to me that she is in reality infinitely better in these respects than we might expect her to be." Mrs. Richards always expressed her gratitude for such suggestions, and then generally said what she pleased.

Nobody could fault American women for a lack of interest in cookery, to be sure—even clubwomen often invited guest speakers to give a presentation on chafing-dish cookery or salad making—but cookery was the very aspect of domestic science that lent itself most often to misinterpretation and greed, or "chocolate cake and lemon pie." During the first decades of the twentieth century, domestic scientists finally declared war on stubborn American women. In September 1899, a few of the domestic scientists most active in the movement, and most distressed by their inadequate public image as mere cooks, called a meeting in order to confront the problem with united action. If the public was unable to grant professional status and respectability to the discipline of housekeeping, then those engaged in the work would grant it to themselves, formally and systematically. The September gathering was the first in a series of ten annual conferences at which domestic scientists worked at carving out a place for themselves among the recognized, academically based professions. Most of the conferences were held at Lake Placid, a resort in upstate New York; at the close of the tenth Lake Placid conference the participants triumphantly declared themselves to be the American Home Economics Association. With this resolution they hoped to bury once and for all the amateur standing of what had been known so widely and casually as domestic science.

The first item of business at the first conference was to choose a new name for the profession. "Domestic science," "household economics," "home science," even the abhorred "household arts" (which suggested mere practical skills rather than scientific principles) were all in use more or less interchangeably at the time, but none seemed just right. The kind of work conveyed by these names, the participants agreed, "could never expect to be recognized as a part of the university curriculum." What they sought was a name that would dictate its own logical placement in the curriculum, in the library, and in the whole arena of human knowledge. Ellen Richards, who presided over the Lake Placid conferences, later summed up the reasoning that led to their final decision. The word "home," she declared, would stand for "the place for the shelter and nurture of children or for the development of self-sacrificing qualities and of strength to meet the world," and "economics" would mean the "management of this home on economic lines as to time and energy as well as to money." There was nothing very radical about this definition—especially its reading of the word "home"—but as a subject heading "home economics" could be inserted right under "economics" and thus would evade any direct link to cooking and cleaning.

In order to make sure that their field, its new name, and its general area of reference were all codified accurately in the realm of knowledge, the Lake Placid group went ahead and chose its own classification in the Dewey Decimal System, Melvil Dewey, who had invented his system of library classification twenty-five years earlier, was a leader in the professionalization of library work and was instrumental in bringing women into what was beginning to be called library science. He and his wife, Annie Dewey, were greatly interested in domestic science, too, and from their summer home at Lake Placid acted as host and hostess for the conferences, as well as being lively participants in the discussions. Originally the Dewey Decimal System had included what it defined as "domestic economy" under the heading Useful Arts, placing it between Agriculture and Communication and Commerce. The women at Lake Placid felt that the heading Useful Arts put too much emphasis on the old-fashioned view of home as a center of production. Women's responsibilities had changed, as Mrs. Richards often pointed out, and the new function of the twentieth-century housekeeper was to consume, to spend money wisely. Home economics would be more appropriately defined under the heading Sociology, they decided, and they selected Number 339 as their own, which placed them between Political Economy and Law. Dewey had assigned Number 339 to another topic—Pauperism—but it seemed plain to the Lake Placid group that pauperism resulted from a "lack of attention to home economics." While the specifics of food, cooking, sanitation, home furnishings, and the like could not be ignored entirely, they could be separated from home economics proper by being kept in their place under Useful Arts. In the classification system as the women finally assembled it, home economics was listed within Sociology and directly under Economics of Consumption, but unfortunately they could come up with only half a dozen subtopics relevant to domestic spending. Most of what happened in the home did belong in Useful Arts, where the subtopics relevant to food alone went on for pages. Eventually Dewey's original scheme, which had the advantage of approximating reality, prevailed in the Dewey Decimal System; but by then the home-economics movement had been safely set on its feet.

Having seized control of their name and, they hoped, their classification, the Lake Placid participants opened battle on what they saw as the most important front: the educational system. Academia had to be the heart of the profession if it was to call itself a profession at all, but in order to penetrate the ranks of higher education, domestic scientists would have to combat a great many wrong impressions of their field. The challenge was immense, and the participants feared that resistance from educational traditionalists would be fierce. "Let us remember we are of one attacking party," a Boston teacher rousingly encouraged her colleagues at the second conference. "All along the line we must storm the defences and plant our standards. It is only by the chance of position that one storms the grammar grades; another battles down the defences of the high school; a third takes the college by assault." One of the most irritating obstacles in their way, as it turned out, was the attitude of some of their own friends and colleagues associated with the Eastern women's colleges. These educators had labored for years to establish at Vassar, Bryn Mawr, Wellesley, and the other select schools a classical curriculum equal to that offered by the best men's colleges. They were deeply reluctant to let domesticity in any guise limit their sense of purpose. Even at Mount Holyoke, where since 1837 students had been required to do a small amount of domestic work in order to keep costs down, President Mary Woolley was trying to persuade students, alumnae, and trustees, who clung to the tradition for sentimental reasons, that the domestic requirement was a waste of students' time. In the continuing struggle to win acceptance for women's higher education, and to prove that women could excel in strenuous academic work, the advocates of domestic science and the advocates of pure classical education had always worked together, and with an appreciable amount of mutual respect. When it came to the question of incorporating course work in domestic science into the college curriculum, however, the women split dramatically.

M. Carey Thomas, the president of Bryn Mawr and a passionate defender of the traditional classical curriculum, told a meeting of the Association of Collegiate Alumnae that she was "astounded" to see vigorous efforts at restructuring that curriculum by including "hygiene, and sanitary drainage, and domestic science, and child-study, and all the rest of the so-called practical studies." Domestic science and sanitation, she stated firmly, "are not among the great disciplinary race studies." They could be pursued after college, she conceded, just as law or medicine or engineering could be pursued, but it was as "preposterous" to compel all women to study domestic science as it would be to compel all men to study dentistry. Mary Roberts Smith, who taught sociology at Stanford, argued just as ardently on the opposite side at another meeting of the ACA. Women had long since proved beyond question that they suffered no mental impairments on account of their sex, Mrs. Smith told her audience. And they had proved beyond question that they could do the same kind of intellectual work that men did. Now they were embarking upon a "third phase" of women's education, in which they would turn to "those lines of thought and scholarship to which their femininity best adapts them. . . ." With no control over her destiny, Mrs. Smith pointed out, a woman could not know whether she would marry, support herself, or engage in charity work. A suitable college curriculum would prepare her at least generally for all of those possibilities. Since most women did marry, domestic training was a necessity—not "cooking or manual training," Mrs. Smith emphasized, but regular study in the "application of pure science to household processes." Mrs. Smith suggested that existing academic departments might easily enlarge their scope to include work pertinent to the home: chemistry and bacteriology, for instance, could perfectly well be taught from the standpoint of the kitchen and sickroom, and the study of economics could be nicely expanded to include women's domestic responsibilities.

At the Lake Placid conferences, countless meetings, discussions, papers, and speeches were devoted to planning just such a massive home-economics syllabus as Mrs. Smith had conjured. What the participants really had in mind was a program that would accompany every girl from kindergarten to postgraduate work, more or less dogging her at every step of her education. By the second conference a Boston teacher had designed a systematic course of study that would begin with hygiene and simple housekeeping in the nursery school, proceed to bacteria and public sanitation in the primary grades, and encompass a new kind of high school—a trade school in home economics—for would-be cooks, parlor maids, and waitresses. College-preparatory high-school students would study chemistry, biology, and physics as usual, but with application to daily life whenever possible. College and graduate work would be devoted to the home from the point of view of economics and sociology, and women could choose their vocations from a range of degree programs including "Home-Maker" and "Social Servant."

The women who spent hours organizing such schemes had in mind the training of citizens, not just cooks or housekeepers, and they had no intention of confining the term "home economics" to the work of a few professionals like themselves. Every woman had the responsibility to run her home intelligently, and every woman could be trained to know the highest and most efficient standards of living. "That is why we plead for the right education of the housewife," Ellen Richards wrote, "not that she shall dust her house, but that she shall know how to infuse into the work that interest and enthusiasm which it has lost owing to circumstances over which she has no control." If the satisfaction of churning butter and weaving cloth was gone from housekeeping, the educated woman could still find in sweeping or dishwashing "a fine action, a sort of religion, a step in the conquering of evil, for dirt is sin." Mrs. Richards often explained that education was more important than income in realizing a successful home—"The cost of living is a mental rather than a material limitation," she told the first Lake Placid conference. And more important than the economics of home life was the ethics of home life. The humblest cottage could be made worthy of her definition of home as the "germ of Anglo-Saxon civilization, the unit of social progress; . . . the nursery of the citizen. . . ."

Shortly after the second Lake Placid conference, one young chemistry teacher who had attended it went to the University of Illinois to set up a new Department of Household Science, in which she hoped to train women citizens according to all the glorious new ideas she had just heard. "I thought I had never seen so flat and so muddy a place: no trees, no hills, no boundaries of any kind," wrote Isabel Bevier, recalling her arrival in Champaign. "This lack of boundaries, physical and mental, the open-mindedness of the authorities and their willingness to try experiments . . . opened up a whole new world to me." Like many of her colleagues, she felt herself to be a pioneer in the wilderness of specialized education for women. She had picked up her own scattered training in chemistry, biology, and nutrition the way many women educated themselves in the sciences: by traveling to whatever places admitted women and working with whatever professors would consent to teach them. It was a chemistry professor in Cleveland, she always remembered appreciatively, who first advised her that the "place for women in chemistry was in work with foods." This mentor foretold a time when the big Midwestern universities "would one day have some kind of a department for foods work with women in it, and I should get ready." Miss Bevier did get ready, by studying with Professor Atwater and doing dietary investigations for him, and by working with Ellen Richards at the Massachusetts Institute of Technology. In the spring of 1900 she received an invitation from the University of Illinois to revive and modernize its long-dormant Ladies Department, housed in the College of Agriculture. That summer she attended the Lake Placid conference, and then, armed with the latest theories, she went on to build a department that quickly became famous as a model of what home economics could be.

Miss Bevier's chief goal was to establish the intellectual pursuit of household science as a serious enterprise—"and thus due warning was given," she wrote, "that neither a cooking school nor a milliner's shop was being opened at the University." Existing courses in architecture and sanitation were moved to the new department and restructured to center on the home, but a greater challenge was to create a program in food study that would not deteriorate into cookery. Examining the catalogues of other state universities that offered "domestic economy," Miss Bevier found that their work in foods was still organized along old-fashioned lines. "The courses were listed as cooking and advanced cooking," she commented disparagingly, "including salads, which I had thought were made mostly from raw materials." Finally she decided her students should approach food as a chemist would, studying each class—proteins, carbohydrates, and fats—in its turn. The term "cooking," Miss Bevier added, "seemed to me so inadequate that after much thought I chose 'selection and preparation of food.'. . ."

The new department opened with twenty students and three courses. Five years later the student body had grown to eighty, and Miss Bevier was offering ten courses for undergraduates and two at the graduate level. Her insistence on a respectable academic foundation for all the course work in her department set Household Science far beyond the usual instruction in cooking and sewing then available at state universities. Course requirements for the B.S. degree in Household Science included botany, bacteriology, zoology, physiology, chemistry, physics, math, design, German, and physical education, as well as special work in household chemistry, domestic bacteriology, domestic architecture, and decoration. Miss Bevier opened an "experimental house" to serve as a laboratory for students working on problems in cooking, furnishing, sanitation, and all the other aspects of domestic management, and remodeled the building according to the most modern ideas in ventilation, lighting, and design. She also outfitted the house with electrical appliances, which themselves drew as many as eighty sightseers a day. In order to keep the purely scientific side of the work firmly in place, she hired a chemist whose sole responsibility was to undertake research in ordinary household processes—"the first woman secured by a department of Home Economics for research work alone," Miss Bevier wrote. "She did outstanding work, finding the answer to the question what makes jelly jell, and also the solutions to many problems regarding bread." When a new president took office at the university, he called in Miss Bevier and inquired with obvious skepticism about the academic qualifications of her students. His assumption was that she was drawing "special students" rather than regularly enrolled degree candidates. This, Miss Bevier wrote, was "too much to stand." She told the president she would check the figures on her enrollments, "and to my joy our proportion of special students was less than that given by the Registrar for the University as a whole." In addition, the president was to learn that Miss Bevier's admission standards for Household Science were much higher than those set for any other department in the College of Agriculture, and that Household Science was the only department in the college that truly functioned at a post-secondary level, according to a rating given by the Carnegie Foundation.

These achievements won the support of the president and the admiration of her fellow home economists, but they aroused the suspicion of a few women in rural Illinois. Miss Bevier shared with the rest of the College of Agriculture a responsibility to spread the word about their work throughout the state, and to help spur the adoption of modern agricultural methods—and modern housekeeping methods—on Illinois farms. Accordingly, she visited private farms, met with the women's division of the state Farmers' Institute, spoke at women's-club meetings, received a constant stream of visitors who were curious to learn "how cooking could belong in a university," and ran a two-week School for Housekeepers every winter, where increasing numbers of local women met for home-economics classes and demonstrations. Miss Bevier's outlook, however, was not received favorably by the sort of local women whom Ellen Richards and Helen Campbell would have lambasted. The women of the state Farmers' Institute were especially hard to convince, for although they, too, were engaged in trying to raise the standards of farm homes, they distrusted Miss Bevier's reliance on experimental and theoretical science to do so. They thought the new department should be a source of practical instruction in housekeeping for anyone who wished to attend, and no more. It was, Miss Bevier wrote, "the age-old conflict between cooking and sewing school adherents and those who believed in the scientific method of approach to the teaching of household science. . . ." Eventually, the opposition from the Farmers' Institute women became so strong that they passed a resolution disapproving of the university's Household Science department. At their instigation, moreover, the experimental house—the showplace of modern laboratory home economics—was closed. Miss Bevier came near to resigning at that point, but because her work was still enthusiastically supported within the university, she was persuaded to stay. Finally, in 1914, the Smith-Lever Act was passed, in effect transferring the work of the Farmers' Institute women—"well-intentioned but uneducational," as Miss Bevier put it—into the hands of trained teachers. This legislation provided funds for extension work, which it defined as "instruction and practical demonstrations in agriculture and home economics," to be given to farm families in their own communities. "It is here that the term *home economics* appears for the first time in federal legislation," Miss Bevier noted with satisfaction. The Smith-Lever Act granted formal acknowledgment to home economics as the necessary parallel to modern agricultural education and rewarded Miss Bevier's efforts with an unmistakable stamp of legitimacy.

By the time of the Smith-Lever Act, the original handful of state university catalogues listing "domestic economy" courses, which Miss Bevier had examined so skeptically when she arrived in Illinois, had grown profusely. Over 250 colleges and universities now offered home economics, with complete four-year programs leading to a B.A. at twenty-eight schools, postgraduate work leading to the master's degree at twenty schools, and a Ph.D. in household administration available at the University of Chicago. In agricultural colleges, in state universities, in technical institutes—in any school where there was coeducation, in fact—departments of home economics were flourishing. Had it not been for coeducation, as Miss Bevier remarked, ". . . it seems as if home economics on a scientific basis would certainly have been delayed for years. . . ." She didn't analyze the reasons, but among the strong supporters of home economics were the presidents of state universities in the West and Midwest, and of private universities like Stanford and the

University of Chicago. These institutions had long been open to women, and the value of female education per se was not in question there. What did give pause to some of these educational leaders was the overwhelming success of their women students. In 1907 President Charles Van Hise of the University of Wisconsin spoke to the Association of Collegiate Alumnae and emphasized what he felt to be some disquieting developments. Women were beginning to equal or outnumber men in liberal-arts courses at the universities, he reported, and they continued to receive higher grades than men, as they had done ever since the start of coeducation. Clearly the admission of women had not brought about a lowering of academic standards in any institution, as had first been feared, Van Hise acknowledged, but there still seemed to be some question as to whether women could do satisfactory work at the graduate level. He suspected, speaking personally, that women did not "incline" to long hours of research. Academic performance aside, Van Hise continued, the presence of women was problematic in another way: they poured into liberal-arts courses in such large numbers that men were beginning to stay away from those subjects. In pre-professional courses such as agriculture or engineering, there were in turn practically no women at all. The solution, as Van Hise and several other presidents saw it, was to follow the trend of this "natural segregation" and institute separate courses for men and women. At the introductory level the courses could be more or less parallel, but at higher levels they should reflect the different interests of the two sexes. Van Hise had no trouble defining several "natural" courses for male study—"engineering, agriculture, commerce, and law"—but then was forced to trail off a bit vaguely, suggesting "other courses, illustrated by home economics, for women. . . ."

Home economics, as it turned out, was sufficient. The idea of coeducation as a parallel system rather than a single track of learning drew notice at many universities where faculty or administration felt overrun by female students. In some schools quotas were established to limit the number of women, and courses were offered in split sections to accommodate men and women separately. By the same token, home economics was able to serve as an academic bulwark against the excesses of coeducation. To home economists themselves, a secure foothold in the university was welcome in any form. At the land-grant institutions, where home economics had grown up as a women's department within the agriculture school, the ideology of parallel training was already in place. "When the boys learn to grow wheat, the girls learn to make it into bread! When the boys raise apples, the girls give them pie!" wrote the founder of the domestic-science program at the Kansas State Agricultural College. "And so both sides of the house shall be trained, until the perfect home shall be attained, and every community will bless those women who are experts in the line of domestic science."

While home economics was not a requirement for women at any of these schools, it was often made especially accessible to the women students by being housed in the same building as the women's gym, the women's dining hall, or the women's dormitory. In addition, home economics enjoyed an unusually fluid position in the university curriculum, so that women ran across it no matter where they concentrated their studies. Its founders always liked to stress the fact that chemistry, biology, economics, art—virtually any academic subject—could be studied profitably from the point of view of the home, and they saw home economics as a natural addition to women's other course work. In some universities it was seen as so natural, in fact, that women who wished to pursue a doctoral degree in one of the sciences were introduced to "special" degree programs combining home economics with their original field. Like Isabel Bevier, who had been told that the place for women in chemistry was in food chemistry, ambitious women were consistently helped to find a place for themselves in home economics. Lita Bane, Miss Bevier's biographer, once wrote the story of her own conversion to home economics, which began when she let her high-school principal know that she wanted to study mathematics in college. The principal warned her that a woman had to be much better than a man to succeed in mathematics and suggested that she try domestic science instead. Miss Bane spent two years, she wrote, "cooking tiny bits of food and making miniature garments," and was ready to quit the field in disgust when she transferred to the University of Illinois and took a course—"a revelation to me"—with Isabel Bevier. "Within a few weeks I found myself saying, 'If this is household science, I'm certainly for it.' She reminded us that the house is not the home as the body is not the Spirit. Yet the house can be made to enhance and enrich home life just as the body can ennoble spiritual life. . . . And to me, the purposes of household science, far from seeming much too petty for college work, now seemed much too large to be encompassed in a four-year course."

The idea of home economics as the women's side of a parallel system, the women's profession in a coeducational world, was a continuing inspiration to believers as well as a comfortable source of institutional support. At the same time, however, home economists were still struggling to disentangle their profession from a welter of tradition and sentiment. Even some of their supporters could not distinguish between scientific domesticity and the old-fashioned kind. When President Charles W. Eliot of Harvard spoke to the Association of Collegiate Alumnae, he urged the creation of a new college curriculum for women, with course work especially suited to their sex and calling. But he was unable to describe that calling in any terms more substantial than "household joy and good." Rhetoric along these lines made the leaders of the movement impatient. "Neither pious intentions nor fulsome oratory about the glories of motherhood . . . furnish an adequate working basis for a serious study of the home," wrote Isabel Bevier in her history of the home-economics movement; she blamed "too much conversation about the 'sphere of woman' as interpreted by men fond of that kind of remark" for holding up progress in the movement early on. Ellen Richards never hesitated to praise the home of the future as a realm of "peace and restfulness and high ideals," but she was equally persistent about the necessity for long, thorough training in science and technology if women were to create such homes. It was no more encouraging for home economists to meet the opposite mentality, however: the women who blindly followed their brothers and took up men's work in offices and shops. Some of these women were suited to business life and some were not, observed a cooking teacher at a meeting of the Cooking Teachers' League. "But of one thing I am certain, that just this woman is needed within the home. And you and I must make it so interesting and attractive to her that she will not want to leave it." What these women lacked, the home economists felt, was the imagination to see beyond cooking and cleaning into the real challenge of modern housekeeping. Neither the sentimentalists nor the new career women seemed to understand that the home had to be confronted with a businesslike attitude hitherto never associated with femininity. Home economics was not a male profession, but it did call for the discipline and the rigorous mental activity of the male professions. Keeping house was not a male responsibility, but it did demand the male mind.

Helen Campbell underscored this point by writing a blunt little story about a women's club that was planning to start a cooking class for the poor. When they met to select a teacher, the club's most ignorant and conservative member spoke up and suggested they hire a certain widow whose fourth and last child had just died. The widow needed the work, and she could hold the class in her own humble kitchen where the pupils would not become confused by modern methods and equipment. It would be a class in pies, doughnuts, and other such products of home cooking; and the very thought of it brought a tear to the clubwoman's eye. "Give me home cooking and the things that mother used to make," she sighed, "about which our dearest associations are entwined." At that, another member of the club sprang up and delivered an angry speech in opposition. "Home cookery!" she cried. "The methods that helped to kill her own children this club will not allow to be applied to others equally helpless. It is a hard thing to say; but the record is plain before us, and I have studied it well." She went on to insist that the club hire a trained teacher, who would use science and nutrition as the basis of instruction. The ignorant clubwoman waited until she finished and then, weeping a bit, resigned from the club, accusing it of abandoning "that reverence for the Home that the true woman must always feel." As she left the room the other member called her an idiot and they all went back to business.

Mrs. Campbell and her colleagues did not deny their own reverence for the home, but they were strict about distinguishing reverence from nostalgia. The "true woman," as they saw her, was no mere creature of tradition; she accepted woman's sphere gladly and then worked to make it a mirror of man's world. Mother's cooking, the old-fashioned country kitchen, the groaning board laden with mince pies—all these familiar symbols of well-being were to them symbols of degeneracy, and the women confined to such a past were doomed. "It was one of these victims who told me that with her own hands she had made in one year twelve hundred and seventy-two pies," Mrs. Campbell reported grimly. "In these houses pie is on tap as it were." The task faced by home economists was to change the focus of domesticity from the past to the future, demolishing the rule of sentiment and establishing in its place the values manifest in American business and industry. American business, in fact, was eager to embrace home economics, and the food industry became a prominent ally in the assault on mother's cooking.

In Homes Like These Crisco is Used
Wherever a housewife takes pride in a clean, sweet kitchen—
Wherever a family insists on food that is wholesome and appetizing—
Wherever a wish for "the best" goes hand in hand with regard for economy—
There Crisco is welcomed and is used with complete satisfaction.

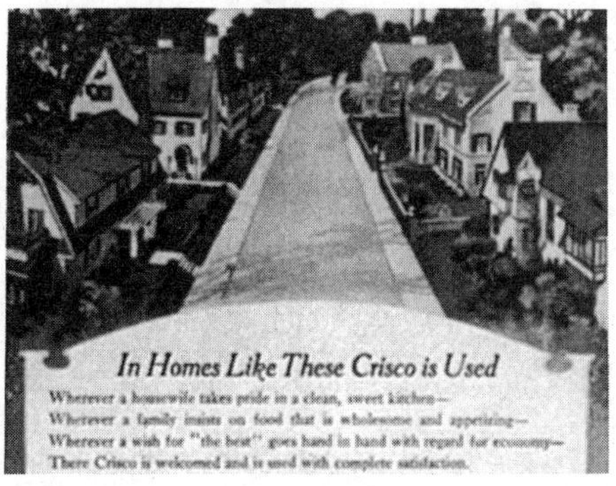

Eight
An Absolutely New Product

We made a canvass of sixty-one poorhouses in thirty-one states, for types of the unsuccessful. We found that ninety-three percent of the inmates were not brought up on oatmeal.

Advertisement for Quaker Oats

A Triumph in Sugar-Making! Sold only in 5 lb. sealed boxes!

Advertisement for Domino Sugar

A dainty dish for luncheon! . . . The most scrupulous care and absolute cleanliness are observed in every process of preparation of this, as well as every one of the other "57 VARIETIES" of HEINZ PURE FOOD PRODUCTS.

Advertisement for Heinz Baked Beans

The pure, high grade, scientifically blended COCOA made by Walter Baker & Co., Ltd. and identified by the trademark of the Chocolate Girl, acts as a gentle stimulant and invigorates and corrects the action of the digestive organs, furnishing the body with some of the purest elements of nutrition.

Advertisement for Baker's Cocoa

In our famous kitchens are many good cooks. They are sorting and soaking—boiling and baking—beans for a million homes. . . . And those beans are the best that were ever baked—in the old times or the new. . . . Home-baked beans cannot compare with

> them, because every home lacks the facilities. Van Camp's are *baked by live steam*. . . . They come out nut-like and whole—not mushy and broken. And all are baked alike. . . . They contain —with the pork—every food element required by the human body.
>
> *Advertisement for Van Camp's Pork and Beans*

> You can hardly find a food in which natural tonic and aperient properties are combined so perfectly with easily-digested nourishment. Surely there never was a prescription more agreeable to "take."
>
> *Advertisement for Campbell's Tomato Soup*

Scientific cookery, both as a cuisine and as a profession, shared the values of the food industry from the outset. During the years in which the cooking schools of Boston, New York, and Philadelphia became established and the cooking-school cooks developed their distinctive cuisine, the technology of food production and the techniques of its distribution were settling into their modern form. Canned goods came onto the market in increasing variety; food that had always been displayed in bulk began to appear in packages; national manufacturers and processors were outstripping, and replacing, local producers; and the use of advertising to gain national recognition for new brand names, new products, and new packages became standard practice. The best-known cooks of the day happily identified themselves with the manufacturers and processors who were applying scientific techniques to food on such a dramatic scale. The manufacturers, in turn, lent the impersonal authority of national industry to the cooking-school cooks. Sarah Tyson Rorer had one of the more active commercial careers: as principal of the Philadelphia Cooking School she had just published her first cookbook when she agreed to join forces with Finley Acker, a Philadelphia grocer whose high-priced retail store displayed the most modern packaged foods and the fanciest imports. In 1886 Acker began publishing *Table Talk*, one of the earliest of the domestic-science magazines. While initially his idea of a useful feature was something called "Grocery News"—several pages of praise for recent achievements in packaging biscuits, olives, jams, and the like—he did invite Mrs. Rorer to contribute more substantially on the subject of food. "Housekeepers' Inquiries," in which she answered readers' questions about cooking and housekeeping, quickly became a popular section of the magazine, and soon Mrs. Rorer was asked to take on two more columns, these slanted forthrightly toward Acker's colleagues in the food business. In "New Things for Table and Kitchen" she applauded various utensils as they arrived on the market, as well as assembling menus and recipes. In "Keystone Dishes" she created a steady supply of whipped, beaten, and aerated desserts and vegetables in honor of a new eggbeater—the "Keystone Beater"—invented by a Philadelphia manufacturing concern. Mrs. Rorer wrote with personality and a commanding style, and her fame grew with the magazine's. Within a year she had started on what would become a subspecialty of her profession: commercial testimonials. "After a *careful and perhaps severe test* of NIAGARA CORN STARCH, I am convinced of its *purity and economy*, and cheerfully recommend it," she stated in one of the first of many such endorsements. In the early years of advertising these endorsements were commonly requested, and granted, without payment. Mrs. Rorer received a supply of Niagara Corn Starch, and the manufacturer gained her stamp of approval, but the important currency to be shared was the public credibility bestowed on both parties by virtue of their association.

After seven years Mrs. Rorer's independent career was assured, and she was able to leave *Table Talk* and start her own magazine, *Household News*. While *Household News* had none of the overt commercialism of *Table Talk*, Mrs. Rorer maintained her personal ties to the food business by continuing to endorse products enthusiastically and by writing numerous "cookbooks" for manufacturers. *Dainty Dishes for All the Year Round* was a collection of frozen desserts and ground-meat entrees, published by a company that made an ice-cream freezer and a meat grinder; and in the same vein Mrs. Rorer wrote *For Serving Shredded Wheat, McIlhenny's Tabasco Sauce Recipes, Recipe Book for the Mudge Patent Processor,* and *Recipes Showing Some of the Many Uses of Wesson Oil.* The activities that kept her reputation thriving were not chiefly these, of course—she had a busy public schedule of teaching and lecturing, and she produced nearly two dozen non-commercial cookbooks—but the food business was an authentic branch of her work and to her way of thinking as respectable as any other branch of it.

Mrs. Rorer's willingness to endorse and promote was shared by the other famous writers and teachers in scientific cookery, and manufacturers made heavy use of their names. "A Bright Galaxy of Stars in the Domestic Firmament Shines Approval on Cleveland's Baking Powder," announced a full-page advertisement in the second issue of *New England Kitchen Magazine.* The names Marion Harland, Mrs. Ewing, Miss Bedford, Mrs. Lincoln, Mrs. Rorer, Mrs. Parker, and Mrs. Dearborn were affixed to seven large stars beaming down upon a can of baking powder. For the most part, such well-known cooks kept their non-commercial writing free of endorsements, but the policy was hardly a rigid one. As early as 1871, Marion Harland was promoting a brand of desiccated codfish in her best-selling manual *Common Sense in the Household,* and Fannie Farmer endorsed a number of products for advertisements that were printed in the back of *The Boston Cooking-School Cook Book.* Editors at *Table Talk* and the *Boston Cooking School Magazine,* in particular, used brand names regularly when they printed two weeks' or a month's worth of daily menus—judging from the casual attitude they exhibited toward the practice, it does not seem to have aroused any controversy. One month the *Boston Cooking School Magazine* ran a recipe for a dessert called Red Robin Pudding and listed the major ingredient as Red Robin wheat. In a later issue a subscriber's query was printed: she wanted to know what Red Robin wheat was, "and where can it be procured?" The magazine answered candidly enough: "We are not familiar with the Red Robin wheat. Think it was a package sent to the school for trial. Any other cereal preparation might be substituted."

Like her colleagues, Mrs. Lincoln was glad to promote what she called "pure food manufacturers," and she never felt the need to justify her links with the food business until she accepted an opportunity to go a bit further and place her name directly upon a baking powder. When Mrs. Lincoln's Baking Powder was introduced, Mrs. Lincoln wrote a long and careful apologia in *American Kitchen Magazine*. "There are many ways in which women may help to give people better food," she began cautiously. Trained cooks might teach, or manage institutions, or cater—"And there are many kinds of business, or manufacturing, especially of pure food products, which might as well be managed by women as by men." She made a point of stating firmly that she had never sold her endorsement of any product, or endorsed anything in which she did not find real merit, and then went on to distinguish this new venture—in which money undoubtedly did change hands—from crude commercialism. "The taste of business life which I have enjoyed in my other work, has aroused an ambition for more, and I prefer it to a life of leisure," she explained. "I see no reason why a woman should not engage in the manufacture of a clean, pure baking powder, as well as in the making of that same powder into cakes or breads and offering them for sale." She would not, she assured her readers, actually go into the factory and grind the powder. But her name and guarantee would appear on the label, and "the highest standard of purity" would be rigorously maintained in the manufacturing process.

Mrs. Lincoln's Baking Powder was a short-lived item, but the kind of good faith Mrs. Lincoln assumed she shared with the manufacturer was emblematic of her profession's trusting attitude toward its commercial counterpart. Her reiterated stress on "pure food products" and "standards of purity" supported an image of the food business as an appropriate place for women in the business world, and it also served as a delicate acknowledgment of the notorious questions that were pressing upon the food business at the time. In 1883 Dr. Harvey Wiley had become head of the Chemical Division at the Department of Agriculture, and he was investigating and publicizing massive evidence of food adulteration. Poisonous chemical preservatives, as well as less harmful adulterants, were constantly being identified in flour, spices, pickles, jams, and numerous other products, including baking powder. Dr. Wiley was campaigning hard for a federal pure-food law, but the food industry managed to avert any federal legislation until 1906. That was the year Upton Sinclair published his graphic descriptions of Chicago meat packing in *The Jungle;* the book aroused such public clamor that Dr. Wiley was at last able to push through his bill. Enforcement was so lax, however, and the wording of the law so generous, that the food industry had little trouble circumventing it.

Meanwhile, the most ardent and vociferous demands for pure food were coming from the food industry itself, which took the position that only a few greedy men dealt in unscrupulous practices, men who were the exceptions in an otherwise upright profession. Moreover, as Finley Acker put it in *Table Talk*, most of the adulterants discovered in food were not "absolutely injurious" but merely cheap substitutions harming the pocketbook more than the person. This was also the attitude of their colleagues in the domestic-science movement, which preferred to treat the issue of food adulteration as an education problem rather than an industrial one, and put a great deal of emphasis on teaching women to shop carefully. Ellen Richards, who had begun the Woman's Laboratory at the Institute of Technology by training her students to perform chemical analyses of the products on the pantry shelf, urged that a "housekeeper's laboratory" be arranged in every home so that women could test for sulphuric acid in the vinegar, ammonia in the baking powder, alum in the bread, and chlorides in the sugar, right in their own kitchens. It was the "average housekeeper" who bore a significant part of the responsibility for food adulteration, admitted a cooking teacher in a paper she presented to the Cooking Teachers' League: too many uneducated housekeepers permitted dealers to sell them cream of tartar that had been extended with rice flour, and pickles and peas that had been colored bright green with copper salts. "The practices which have savored of dishonesty on the part of some dealers have had their origin through the ignorance of the consumer," declared an editorial in *New England Kitchen Magazine*. Once women knew enough to insist upon pure foods and refused to buy all others, these teachers believed, the handful of manufacturers involved in serious food adulteration would find that it did not pay.

Dedicated as they were to enlightening the ignorant and conservative housekeeper, scientific cooks greeted with acclaim the traveling food expositions that toured the nation in the 1890s. These "pure food fairs" were organized by the major food companies in an effort to counter the adulteration scandals with a more favorable public image of the industry, and they attracted huge crowds. The manufacturers would set up lavishly decorated booths displaying their products, selling a portion for a few pennies or offering free samples. Along with the commercial display, the exhibitors would present a series of public lecture-demonstrations on cookery, drawing upon local cooking schools for lecturers or importing one of the nationally known cooks to speak. Sarah Tyson Rorer added an enterprising sideline to her career by traveling around the country with one of the expositions, setting herself up in each new hall just like the Quaker Oats display or the Horlick's Malted Milk, and giving lectures at every stop. In cities such as Boston and Philadelphia, where the cooking establishment was especially vigorous, local domestic scientists would arrange extensive educational programs to accompany the exposition, scheduling lectures, creating model kitchens, and displaying thematic table settings. The entire phenomenon—America's most important food businesses, the exemplars of modern production and packaging, arrayed in a massive hall, with distinguished cooks holding forth and throngs of people in attendance—thrilled the domestic scientists. At these moments the food industry took on for them the glory of the Crusades.

> One could not gaze upon the novel, artistic and expensive exhibits and note the names of the exhibitors—names which are household words throughout the length and breadth of our land, and some of them familiar to the eye and ear of the whole of Christendom—without a feeling of profound admiration for the sagacity, the pluck, and indomitable perseverance of the men who have, by sheer force of intellect and energy, placed everywhere at the hand of the consumer, wholesome food products, and at a price within the command of our most humble citizens [wrote a correspondent at the Chicago Pure Food Exposition to *New England Kitchen Magazine*].

The Philadelphia exposition of 1892 was typically resplendent, and since it was sponsored by a grocers' association headed by Finley Acker, it received bountiful coverage in *Table Talk.* According to the *Table Talk* reporter, Industrial Hall was draped with American flags, bunting, and wreaths, and throughout the exposition Mark Hassler's Orchestra "flooded the building with sweet sounds." Among the more noteworthy booths was the Pettijohn's Breakfast Food display, which featured a life-size wax sculpture of a woman in riding habit next to a horse, both of them surrounded by sheaves of wheat and oats. Another life-size wax woman could be viewed at the Pearline booth, makers of soap; this figure—"evidently by birth and profession a scrubber, clad in coarse working-dress"—held Pearline in her hand "and laughed that she had found a friend." Real women were the motif at the Baker's Chocolate booth, where cups of cocoa were handed around by "chocolate maidens" dressed to imitate the trademarked picture on the box. At the Purity Dried Fruit display, vine leaves and clusters of grapes were hung about the booth. *Table Talk* remarked that every woman "smiled with approval in passing this exhibit. To wash currants is one thing, to buy them beautifully clean, in a neat compact package, is quite another and more acceptable method."

Equally ingenious displays were organized for a Boston exposition that opened two years later, filling a six-acre exhibition hall and hailed by its sponsors as the World's Food Fair. A miniature margarine factory was set up on one countertop, and a salt company earned the "palm of originality," according to *New England Kitchen Magazine*, for constructing its booth entirely from bags of salt. A towering chimney of baking-powder cans was the centerpiece of the Cleveland Baking Powder display; at its base was a stove where cooks produced a continuing procession of baking-powder biscuits and cakes. Elsewhere on the floor a cereal machine was in operation all day long, transforming whole grains into shredded wheat, and an electrically operated dairy churned up to 3,000 pounds of butter every day. Swift and Company, the Chicago meatpacking house not yet made notorious by Upton Sinclair's exposé, had what *New England Kitchen Magazine* called a "dainty" booth, decorated with puffs of pink-and-white muslin. On hand to greet the public at the Swift display were "young lady attendants in pretty gowns of pink, always wearing white flowers and seeming to be a part of the picture."

The wholehearted admiration expressed by domestic scientists for these elaborate advertising tableaux—"Surely a philanthropic work—a sort of 'life-saving service' on land," in the view of *Table Talk*—was more than a reflection of their commercial ties to the industry, it was an open bow to some of their most respected coworkers. *New England Kitchen Magazine* did concede that the "business adventurer" intent on making money had been one of the first to take advantage of food expositions, but the magazine believed that such men had been quickly replaced by "honest and intelligent" dealers, who joined with the "social missionaries" of scientific cookery to lift the exhibitions onto a thoroughly educational level. By rights it was the "social missionaries" from local cooking schools who had charge of the cookery lectures and demonstrations. When these became as extensive as they did in Boston, the local domestic scientists were enormously proud to acknowledge that they were equal partners with the food industry, awakening the public to the issue of food and reaching thousands "who perhaps would never attend a cooking school." Lectures on cookery took place every morning at the World's Food Fair, and they were followed every afternoon and evening by more lectures on related topics, among them "The Art of Entertaining," "Water and Ice Supply," "Bacteria as Friends and Foes," and "Dust and Its Dangers." A model bedroom—"dainty and beautiful and at the same time sanitary," applauded *New England Kitchen Magazine*—was on display. Carrie Dearborn of the Boston Cooking School arranged a series of decorative table settings on themes including "Edible Flowers," "A Dietetic Luncheon," and "A Japanese Ceremonial Tea." Every day at noon there was a Hygienic Lunch, with a visiting expert in hygienic living presiding at the table; these featured a great many boiled and scalloped vegetables, with no meat, butter, or salt. A teacher from the Boston Cooking School made an additional series of Economic Lunches, using the Aladdin Oven, and other experts from the Boston Cooking School contributed their specialties—one organizing a Tennis Tea, and another setting up a Rosebud Luncheon. " 'Say, is this the harvest supper or what?' said someone, looking at the little tables arranged for the 'Five o'clock Tea.' " *New England Kitchen Magazine* found it very amusing that so many people at the fair were bewildered by the cookery displays. One man, the magazine reported, examined the "Mermaid's Dinner" and decided it was an oyster supper; somebody else took a look at "the dainty platters of fillets of halibut and chicken timbales" and identified the whole array as ice cream. "Surely these expositions but open the way for schools of domestic science," the magazine concluded with satisfaction.

The sense of high purpose that scientific cooks felt they shared with the food industry turned these food expositions into symbols of collegiality and mission. The cooking-school graduates who worked as attendants in many of the booths, preparing baking-powder biscuits or dressing up in costume to pass out samples of hot chocolate, heralded a new factor in the food business, as *New England Kitchen Magazine* saw it—"the influence of the cooking schools." Already graduates were being employed by food manufacturers to demonstrate products and create recipes, and increasingly the association between commercial and non-commercial cookery seemed as natural as it was intimate. "Once more we are asked to give notice to the closing of a food exposition," wrote Sarah Tyson Rorer in *Household News*, as one exposition concluded its stay in Cleveland and prepared to move on to Detroit. "These closing notices come to us almost like notices of dying friends." Such products as Knox Gelatin, Snider Catsup, Armour Beef Extract, and Hecker's Self-Rising Flour—all of them habitually on display at the expositions—presented themselves as the future of American cookery in terms that wholly supported the ideals of domestic science. Uniformity, sterility, predictability—the values inherent in machine-age cuisine—were always at the heart of scientific cookery, so the era of manufactured and processed food descended upon the domestic-science movement like a millennium. In the physical achievements of processing—the sanitary gloss, the smooth, unvarying texture, the evenness of quality—it was possible to see the technological equivalent of white sauce. At the conclusion of a series of articles on cheese ("From Cottage and Cave"), Mrs. Lincoln compared the American product with the foreign varieties and had no difficulty arriving at a preference. American factory cheese, she stressed, was a composite: the milk was gathered from different areas and mixed together, so the resulting cheese lacked the "individuality" that characterized foreign cheeses. "Those who can remember the great diversity in taste, structure, and composition which was so noticeable in the old farmhouse cheeses can appreciate the greater uniformity in the factory product," she went on. "The method is more economical of material, time, and labor; it removes this burden from our farming women; neatness and cleanliness are obligatory; the quality of the product can be gauged and assured, and the cost and trouble of marketing are greatly lessened."

With the help of the new industry of advertising, the food business was able to reflect Mrs. Lincoln's values perfectly, by keeping its achievements in packaging, sanitation, convenience, and novelty at the forefront. The message constantly projected by the food business was that technology was transforming food, and for the better, a message that progressive women were glad to believe. According to the industry, for example, canned foods were not only convenient, they were an improvement. "A dainty dish for luncheon!" was the banner headline on an advertisement for Heinz baked beans. This was a daring claim, since baked beans, while popular, had never been classed as a "dainty" food. Sarah Tyson Rorer went so far as to forbid brain-workers to eat them even once a week —no literary person, she said, could digest baked beans. It was the can that made the difference. As later ads explained, the thoroughness and sterility of factory baking changed beans into an appropriate, completely digestible dish for men, women, and children, in all seasons. The ultimate in the reclassification of baked beans was reached when an anonymous cook employed by the Snider Company took a can of Snider's Pork and Beans, mixed the contents with celery, onions, salad dressing, and whipped cream, and called it a Bean Celery Salad. In the same fashion, other canned foods were boosted to a higher culinary station. At first canned fruits and vegetables had been seen largely as emergency foods, useful when nothing else was at hand. "No person would claim that canned foods are to be chosen when fresh ones are available, but the ease in keeping them and quickness of preparation are great advantages at times," Anna Barrows conceded in 1898. A decade and a half later a food writer announced in a magazine that canned fruits and vegetables had so improved in quality that they were now preferable to fresh produce, unless the housekeeper had her own garden and orchard and was regularly putting up her supplies. ("Lucky is she among women, but she is in the decided minority.") In the process of canning peas, she emphasized,

> hands do not come into direct contact with the pea through all its progress from the vine to the table. . . . Only recently have machines been put on the market which husk corn and cut it from the cob so that this, too, escapes handling. The beets which are canned in various sizes are topped, sorted, boiled, the skins rubbed off, and they are put into cans by machinery. . . . The advantages offered by all these processes in preserving food in perfect cleanliness cannot be overlooked by the housekeeper who struggles to keep her kitchen and its contents free from dirt, germs, and consequent disease.

Moreover, she told her readers, the speed with which vegetables were gathered and canned was enough to ensure their perfect freshness—her own family declared them more delicious than the produce she had purchased formerly.

Somewhat unconvincingly, the writer also stated that she was not setting down these thoughts "with the intention of pushing the interests of the makers of canned foods." By the time she was writing, in 1914, it hardly mattered whether or not a food expert was actually employed by the industry. As advertising became a more crucial factor in the economics of magazine publishing, food columns increasingly reflected commercial interests, and scientific cookery itself settled comfortably into the service of the industry. Food ideas that were developed in the company kitchen, and food ideas that sprang from the independent experts, were so compatible that together they set in motion what both had desired: a single cuisine for all of middle-class America. New products, new methods, and new combinations were quickly absorbed into the teaching of the most famous cooks and home economists, whose culinary imaginations were well primed.

One commercial ingredient that was swept into prominence during this era was tomato catsup, for the blunt, sweet flavor and the certainty of the results made it highly popular with scientific cooks. As a housekeeper in one of the advertisements put it, " 'Why, we never make a brown gravy and scarcely a soup but what we put in a little Snider's Tomato Catsup. It is much easier than taking a little of this and a little of that and then, maybe, never having things twice alike. The Catsup is always the same, and gives a flavor that everyone seems to like, so it is always a safe seasoning.' " Thinking very much the same way, the food editor who replaced Sarah Tyson Rorer at *Table Talk* habitually listed "beefsteak tomato ketchup" in her daily menus. Mrs. Rorer, who had gone to *Household News*, combined catsup with sherry to sauce some leftover veal. Half a cup of tomato catsup thickened with flour was Mrs. Lincoln's choice of a gravy suitable for fricasseed partridges, and in July 1911, it was Fannie Farmer who brightened up a French dressing by stirring a spoonful of catsup into it.

The characteristic sweetness of much American cooking was also established during these years, as cooks relied more and more on the blandness and general acceptability of sugar as a flavoring. Canned pineapple, sugared grapefruit, marshmallows, and flavored gelatins found new and sometimes dazzling roles in the menus and recipes constructed around these increasingly popular ingredients. On a hot summer evening dinner might begin, as the *Boston Cooking School Magazine* suggested, with an appetizer of lemon gelatin that had been poured into a banana skin containing, instead of its banana, four carefully made banana balls. "When opened the banana looks like a mammoth yellow pea pod," the magazine said encouragingly. For teatime there was a baked cream-cheese-and-marshmallow sandwich, and for an unspecified occasion, grapefruit halves bordered with maraschino-flavored whipped cream and glacéd cherries. More than any other part of the meal, however, it was the salad course that was expanding most rapidly in size and splendor under the influence of the new ingredients. Two of the more important variations were introduced by Fannie Farmer, who livened up her Los Angeles Fruit Salad—a mixture of canned pineapple, grapes, and walnuts—by adding pieces of marshmallow, an innovation in gratuitous sweetening that was remarkable even by her own standards. Then, creating a gelatin salad for a ladies' luncheon menu to be printed in *The Woman's Home Companion*, she added a cup of ginger ale to the gelatin mixture and folded in some cut-up grapes, celery, apples, and pineapple. She called it, modestly, a fruit salad—but the famous Ginger Ale Salad had been born. Meanwhile, as salads like these edged closer to dessert, the sweet course itself was gaining in extravagance. Desserts had never been a particularly subtle feature of American cooking, but with the advent of sheer sweetness as a virtue they became formidable. Even gingerbread, a humble favorite for well over a hundred years, was spruced up for the new century with a filling of melted marshmallow. The same treatment was considered appropriate for ice cream, another of the nation's great traditional desserts. According to the *Boston Cooking School Magazine*, this old-fashioned treat could be improved by freezing plain ice cream with melted marshmallows, and then adding chopped marshmallows to the result. The sweetest and most garish of the reconstructed desserts were the ones with the most fragile names—Angel's Food, or Ecstasy Dessert, or Heavenly Pudding. These combined marshmallows, candied fruit, macaroons, white cake, gelatin, and whipped cream in one fashion or another, sometimes with the addition of pink food coloring. "I usually go in for the substantials in life, yet occasionally frills prove necessary," apologized a Cambridge home economist who was contributing a recipe for pink Angel Food to a progressive cookbook. The dessert, she promised, would provide "new stomach sensations."

Under the powerful combined influence of the educators and the food industry, the nation's eating habits became identifiably American. The extraordinary degree of predictability that was the triumph of mass-produced food had been sought for years by laboratory-based scientific cooks, and its achievement represented the fulfillment of one of the major goals in domestic science: the attainment of certainty. An ever-sturdier sense of finitude, objectivity, and perfect control could now be discerned in recipes and meal plans that professional cooks sent forth from schools and manufacturers. Sometimes, in fact, it was possible for a cooking teacher to strip away so much of what she considered extraneous to the process of cookery that the remainder could be reduced to a chart, itself a stunning acknowledgment of the now frozen distance that separated the cook from the food. Those who admired them were continually being misled by the magic of charts, as if the imposition of headings, subheadings, ruled lines, and neat boxes really could subdue all that remained stubbornly uncontrollable in the kitchen. The director of cooking classes at a New York school took great pride in her cake diagrams, which were meant to show how a plain cake (No. 1) could be changed to a cake with raisins, nuts, chocolate, etc. (No. 2), or to a completely different cake (No. 3). A child who mastered this diagram to the extent of being able to reproduce it using three-eighths of a cup of flour was then permitted to bake a "small specimen" as a reward. Another, more elaborate cake chart was produced by a cook employed by the United Gas Improvement Company to promote the use of gas stoves. *Choice Receipts—Arranged for the Gas Stove* was a small cookbook decidedly belonging, as *New England Kitchen Magazine* said, to the modern era. All the recipes were as condensed and simplified as the author could make them, and in her section on cakes she managed to provide nearly fifty recipes in fewer than five pages. The chart for cupcakes alone supplied twenty-eight varieties. Seven spice cakes and eleven sponge cakes

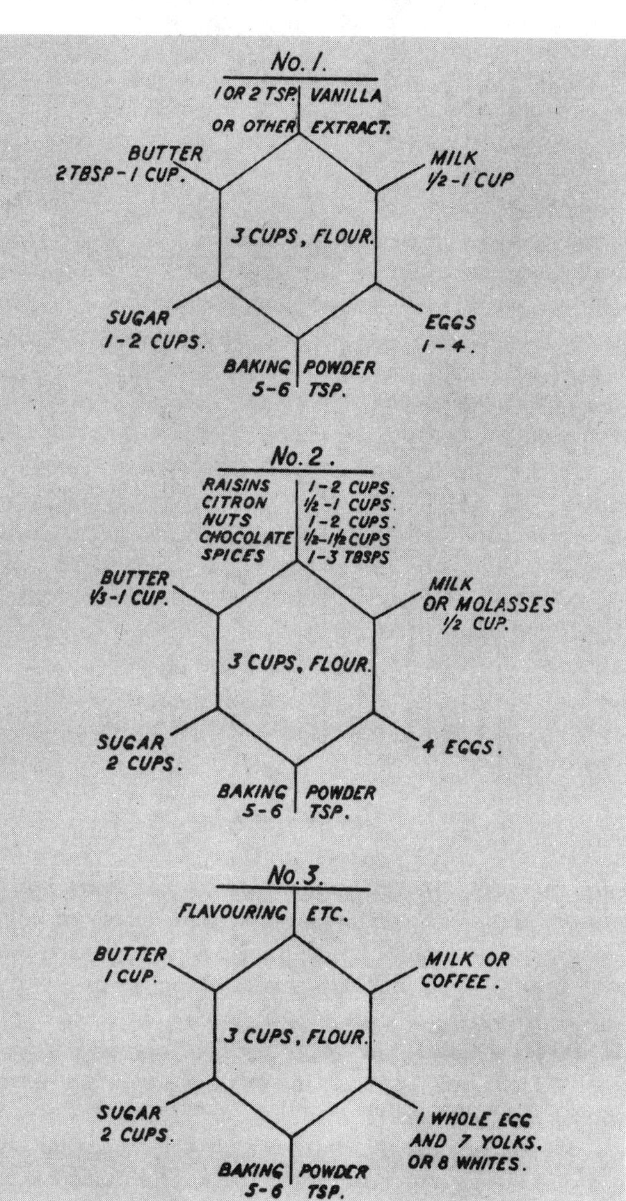

Cake Diagram

C. Butter.	C. Sugar.	C. Flour.	T. Bp.	Whites of Eggs.	Yolks of Eggs.	C. Milk.	FLAVORING.
¼	1	1½	1½	1	1	½	Yellow rind of 1 lemon.
¼	1¼	2½	2½		2	1	One t. lemon juice.
¼	1	2	2	2	2	1	1 t. vanilla.
¼	1	1	1	2	2	¼	1 oz. chocolate melted.
¼	1	1½	1½	3		½	Rose.
¼	1	2	2	4		¾	½ c. chopped nuts.
¼	1½	2½	2	2	3	1	
¼	1½	2	2	6		½	½ t. Almond extract.
¼	1	1½	2		8	½	1 t. Lemon juice.
⅓	1½	2½	2	2	6	½	1 t. Lemon juice.
½	1½	2	1½	4		1	
½	2	3	2	2	3	1	
½	2	3	2	2	4	1	
½	1	2	2		6	½	1 t. Lemon juice.
½	2	2	1½	6		¾	
½	2	3	3	3	3	½	
½	1¼	2	2	3	3	½	
½	2	3	2	8		¾	Pistachio.
½	2	3	2	4	4	1	
½	1	1½	2		8	½	1 t. Lemon juice.
⅔	2	3	2	3	3	1	
¾	1½	2¼	2	3	3	½	
¾	2	3	2	1	6	1	
¾	2	3⅓	3	3	6	1	1 t. Lemon juice.
1	2	3	2	4	4	1	
1	3	3¼	3	4	4	1	1 Grated cocoanut.
1	2	3	3	8		1	½ t. Almond extract.
1	3	4	3	12		1	1 Lemon, 1 c. citron.

Cupcake Chart

were presented in the same fashion, and directions for mixing, along with other pointers, were added in concise paragraphs attached to each table. Awkward as it would have been to read and follow such "recipes" in the actual course of making a cake, the author's success in keeping the messy business of food and cookery well removed from its scrupulously systematic image won the admiration of her colleagues.

Nearly two decades later the pristine appeal of charts was still strong, inspiring the director of domestic science in the Washington, D.C., public schools to diagram the nutritional components of an entire eating plan for three days. Addressing a group of housekeepers in Baltimore in

1911, Emma Jacobs arranged three "Typical Correctly Balanced Menus" on a chart, planning them for a hypothetical man weighing 154 pounds, with good digestion. Balance was the most important factor by far in these model menus, so protein, carbohydrate, and fat were distributed with an exactitude that demanded kitchen scales, a ruler, and some arithmetic. Atop two breakfast rolls, for example (combined weight, two ounces; cost, two cents; percent protein, .170; calories, 163), the man was permitted to spread a one-inch cube of butter (weight, one ounce; cost, two and a quarter cents; percent protein, none; calories, 224). Every morsel of every meal for three days was specified—"8 steamed dates," "4 or 6 leaves lettuce"—and Miss Jacobs advised her audience to apportion daily nutrients to their families on the basis of equally precise calculations. What eluded her scrutiny, however, was the nature of the food itself. To balance a meal by numbers alone, ignoring taste and texture, meant that creamed potatoes, creamed vegetable soup, macaroni with cream sauce, salad with a creamy dressing, and gelatin with cream were all listed on the menu for Day Two, along with stewed prunes, stewed corn, and stewed tomatoes. The one-inch cube of butter deemed sufficient for two breakfast rolls on Day One was reduced the next day at dinner to a half-inch cube for three slices of bread, because the amount of fat already included in the meal made the second half inch redundant, yet the bread was needed for the carbohydrate total. Again a half cube of butter appeared on the breakfast menu for Day Three, this time reduced on account of the sausage at the same meal. But with three slices of toast and a quarter cup of "coarse hominy" allotted as well, half an inch of butter would not have had much effect on an exceedingly dry portion of carbohydrates that morning. Two ounces of stewed prunes were assigned to help.

Graphs and charts never did make their way into daily use in ordinary kitchens, but the state of mind they projected—impersonal and absolutely assured—became increasingly attractive to modern housekeepers. The profession of home cook, which had been launched with microscopes and chemistry texts and a fever of analysis, was beginning to rise into the loftier, more general role of home manager, just as Ellen Richards had foreseen when she wrote "Housekeeping in the Twentieth Century." The era of efficiency was on its way. As the old-fashioned kitchen was reduced in size and function until it became the kitchenette, more than one reformer was happy to predict that it was about to disappear entirely. Surveying the abundance of canned foods, packaged biscuits and cereals, cooked meats, prepared salads, and bakery goods available at the start of the new century in 1900, a group of college-educated Boston women decided that "home cooking as we now know it" would soon be a thing of the past, at least for city dwellers. In the interests of hastening this process, they invited a Wellesley graduate to conduct a series of experiments in the comparative cost of home-cooked and ready-made foods, hoping to prove by the superiority of the latter that it was already time for "conservative home-makers" to accept the inevitable course of industry. Bread, stuffed turkey, stuffed fowl, and finally three whole days' worth of meals were tested, the method being first to prepare the food at home and then to purchase the same articles from a bakery, a delicatessen, or the New England Kitchen. In all cases, unfortunately, the results were discouraging: the people tasting both products preferred the homemade food, and it cost less. Nonetheless, these progressives stood firm in their belief that manufactured and pre-cooked foods were the way of the future. The fact that baker's bread was distinctly inferior to the homemade, for example, they attributed to the lack of a "common and accepted 'standard' of what really good bread is." When such a standard was articulated there would be a "general demand" for better bread, and bakers would comply. In the meantime, they noted, most bakeries produced bread at least as acceptable as that made by the average, unscientific home cook. Similarly, they refused to be swayed by the failure of the three days' worth of pre-cooked meals. The problem seemed to be with some dishes more than others—cooked eggs, soufflés, "all the dishes which spoil by standing, or which depend upon immediate serving for their peculiar delicacy"—and they felt that a more limited menu of soups and stews would have won better favor.

The truly prophetic aspect of this experiment was the ease with which the Boston group glided over questions of taste, freshness, and quality. These women—who had no commercial affiliations but were active in local reform organizations and fired with the spirit of the age—were ready for the new rule of efficiency, ready for the kitchen that ran itself. The kind of cookery suitable for the century they awaited was a set of procedures carried out without waste or distraction, an event in which every whim was eliminated, every challenge deflected, and every question obviated. In the *Home Science Cook Book*, written by the editors of *New England Kitchen Magazine* as a summing up of their methods and experience, even the role of fancy cookie cutters was reduced to the pragmatic: when half a batch of cookies had been flavored with lemon, and the other half with coconut, then and only then might two different shapes reasonably be used to avoid confusion. At the same time, however, such a carefully maintained impersonality between the cook and the food meant that the most alarming culinary disruptions and innovations were allowed on the dinner table as long as they behaved themselves. Neatness, order, and functionalism were commanded just as well by a frosting sandwich—which the *Boston Cooking School Magazine* suggested for a child's lunch box—as by jelly or chopped egg. And when the same magazine recommended that glacé cherries be soaked in sherry and poured over sautéed tenderloin steak, the overwhelming results could be interpreted as a festive variation on pork with applesauce, or turkey with cranberries. Scientific cookery had always been marked by a comfortable swing between the drab and the bizarre; indeed, the very same cooking teacher who believed in cutting the lettuce into uniform strips for tidiness went on to create a salad made of sliced bananas and pimentos covered with mayonnaise and whipped cream. No matter how insistently serious-minded they were, the most popular scientific cooks could accept novelty as progress.

By 1913, the year Woodrow Wilson was inaugurated, the meals evolved from scientific cookery had come to dominate a great deal of formal and institutional catering, as well as many home kitchens; the food was familiar to Americans everywhere. At the end of Wilson's first day in office, in fact, he and his guests were served a dinner so orderly, so white, and so creamy it might have been planned at cooking school. It included cream of celery soup, fish with white sauce, roast capon with two white vegetables (cauliflower and mashed potatoes), a fruit salad, and a dessert made with gelatin, custard, and whipped cream. The livelier tastes and traditions that still flourished in immigrant families and communities were supplying the nation with more adventurous perspectives on food, but scientific resistance was strong. "Americans do not as a rule take to these foreign foods . . . although some of the best have been popularized and adopted," claimed a contributor to *American Kitchen Magazine*, which titled the article "Queer Foreign Foods in America." The immigrant tended to prefer the "food of his fatherland," the article noted, "even though coarse and unsavory compared with the food of his adopted land." A few of the scientific cooks, notably Sarah Tyson Rorer and Helen Campbell, did express enthusiasm for certain kinds of foreign cookery—Mrs. Rorer liked Indian and Sinhalese curries, which she learned to make from the South Asian representatives at the 1893 World's Fair, and Mrs. Campbell praised the "Hindoo" way with vegetables. But even those who were fascinated with strange dishes hesitated to step very far inside new territory. Mrs. Rorer's directions for Chinese Eggs resulted in a serving of hard-boiled eggs with white sauce, and a "Japanese luncheon" detailed by the *Boston Cooking School Magazine* featured bean sprouts with hollandaise sauce. One of the most wholeheartedly appreciative reports on foreign cookery came from a man who visited a Japanese restaurant in Seattle and wrote up his experiences for *American Kitchen Magazine*. For only ten cents he had eaten a delicious meal, and he commended the proprietor, the cooks, and the waiters for their "intellectual merits" and good work habits. A second meal at the restaurant was pronounced just as good, and with the exception of a certain plate of vegetables—"which I have not yet had the courage to test"—he carefully described the different dishes he had ordered, namely a steak, some fried potatoes, bread and butter, milk, a roll, and a bowl of oatmeal.

European cookery aroused much less suspicion than Asian, of course, but in general the conversion of foreign foods into American dishes was carried out by blunting the flavors and dismantling the complications. The cooking magazines frequently did run recipes for German salads or French soups, and the reformers were constantly urging Americans to eat more lentils and macaroni as inexpensive forms of protein; but as far as these cooks were concerned, the truly important culinary innovations of the day were the ones that promoted a greater degree of dietary standardization. One participant at the fourth Lake Placid conference had taken an informal poll of twenty-two families to find out what they ate, and the results distressed her. Although there was a great deal of repetition in the daily menus within each household, she told her colleagues, the variety from house to house was dizzying. Evidently "local tastes and family idiosyncrasies" still exerted a powerful influence over the dinner table, preventing the development of "conscious standards" in meal planning. "We need to learn the meaning of *democracy in taste* in regard to food . . ." she pleaded. "The 'breaking of bread' is a universal sacrament and it is given to men primarily for the strengthening of their bodies, not for the gratification of their palates. To make the choice of food a matter of whims and unreasoning habit . . . —is this not to forget the first law of social righteousness, 'Man shall not live unto himself alone'?"

Another expert at the same conference pointed reassuringly to "the great bakeries, canning factories and creameries" as welcome signs of progress toward centralization in food preparation, an industrial development that was certain to lead to "democracy in taste." Unlike those few traditional industries that lent pride and satisfaction to the individual worker and for that reason deserved to remain in private hands—fine bookbinding was her example—cookery was essentially a mechanical, repetitive task, and thus perfectly suited to mass production. Even more important, she emphasized, the need for food was the same in everyone. "Scientists tell us that all healthy people with the same amount of exercise need the same quantity of food of the same composition," she explained. "It is true that all people do not demand the same kind of food. This is due sometimes to acquired appetites, sometimes to finicalities of appetite due to bad living and sometimes to the fact that people have not enough other interests besides that in eating and drinking." When people advanced to the stage of what she called "rational living"—"plenty of exercise in the fresh air, with work that leads to physical, mental and spiritual development"—they would find that "unreasonable preferences for particular foods" disappeared. Appetite, like nutritional requirements, would be alike in everyone.

Those innovations in American eating habits that began in a manufacturer's laboratory, passed into the hands of home economists, and then met the public by way of the advertising industry took root with a speed and sureness that gratified the most forward-looking cooks. The campaign to place Crisco in every kitchen was a model of the process, and Crisco itself was in many ways a model food of the twentieth century. "An Absolutely New Product," announced one of the introductory advertisements. "A Scientific Discovery Which Will Affect Every Kitchen in America." Crisco had been tested extensively in the laboratory ever since its discovery, the copy explained, and "chefs and domestic science teachers" had been using it experimentally as well. Now it was ready for the public: "Dip out a spoonful and look at it. You will like its very appearance, for it is a pure cream white, with a fresh, pleasant aroma." Its advantages over butter were numerous, according to the manufacturer, for butter could melt or spoil, it changed from season to season, and its origins were often unsanitary. "Crisco never varies," the copy stressed. "Crisco is never sold in bulk, but is put up in immaculate packages, perfectly protected from dust and store odors. No hands touch it. . . ."

Crisco did not replace butter or even lard as extensively as the manufacturer had planned, but it was incorporated into a great deal of cookery readily enough, with a loss of flavor that ranged from inconsequential to revolutionary. At first the recipes created by experts like Janet McKenzie Hill, who edited the *Boston Cooking School Magazine* and was hired to write one of the first Crisco cookbooks, concentrated mostly on the unexceptional use of Crisco in pastry, baking, and frying. Later, however, the manufacturer began to commandeer and publish a greater variety of standard recipes. Caramel Sweet Potatoes could be glazed with brown sugar and Crisco; stuffed onions could be filled with bread crumbs and Crisco; sandwiches could be spread with Crisco mixed with an egg yolk and seasoned rather highly with Worcestershire sauce, lemon juice, and vinegar; and finally, a pure and tasteless white sauce could be prepared by melting two tablespoons of Crisco, adding two tablespoons of flour, and stirring in a cup of milk.

With the Crisco white sauce, scientific cookery arrived at a food substance from which virtually everything had been stripped except a certain number of nutrients and the color white. Only a cuisine molded by technology could prosper on such developments, and it prospered very well. So did the home cook, in one way, for as prepared foods took over the kitchen, her culinary success came to be measured in conviction, not skill. Between World War I and the 1960s, generations of women were persuaded to leave the past behind when they entered the kitchen, and to ignore what their senses told them while they were there. "The final goal," Isabel Bevier used to advise her would-be chemists and nutritionists at the University of Illinois when the school year was over, "is gracious womanhood." With this benediction, the taming of food was complete.

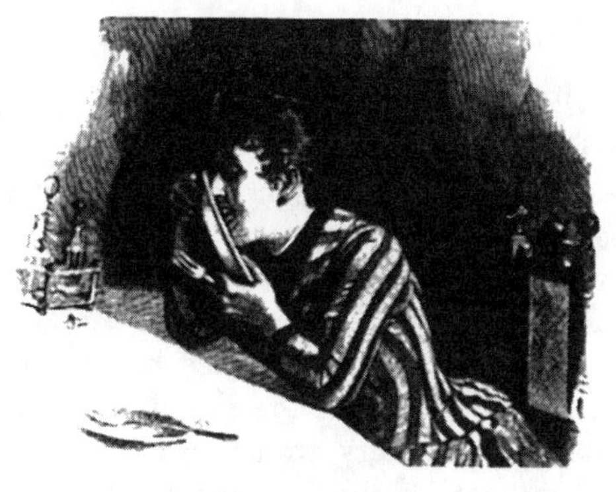

Conclusion
A Leaf or Two of Lettuce

I have only made carrot-and-raisin salad once, the day it was taught to me in seventh grade, but the memory of those bright orange shreds specked with raisins and clotted with mayonnaise has been unaccountably hard to shake. It's easy to understand why the recipe appealed to the teacher—carrots made it nutritious, raisins made it sweet, and mayonnaise made it a salad—but I can't explain why a combination I never hoped to eat again was able to lodge itself so firmly into the apparatus of my adolescence. Perhaps those endless Wednesday-afternoon classes, known by 1958 as "Homemaking," had a grip on us that we hardly suspected at the time, codifying as they did a grim and witless set of expectations that loomed across the future like a ten commandments for girls. Eerily enough, this course, which purported to be about the real world, had nothing whatever to do with anything that happened in my home or that I had ever seen happen anywhere else. Why were they claiming life was like this? Who on earth wore pink cotton "hostess aprons" or, worse yet, had to sew them? None of us knew enough to rebel in those days, but the sheer emptiness at the core of home economics was stunning, if not within the reach of consciousness just then.

Ellen Richards, Sarah Tyson Rorer, even Isabel Bevier never dreamed of a future so vacuous, never suspected that the profession they designed to reign over the new century would grow feeble almost as soon as the new century touched it. Domestic science had been a reform movement: its focus was on the grand and possible, and its assessment of ordinary women was impatient. With a healthy disrespect for the past and a relentless commitment to human perfectibility, the leaders of the movement set about cleansing, renewing, and redirecting. Theirs was the energy born of dissatisfaction—what they saw just wasn't good enough; they wanted to make it better. To question the certainty of woman's domestic fate was beyond the scope of the movement. But within the boundaries of the household revolution as domestic scientists conjured it, the importance of inquiry, criticism, and change were paramount. Increasingly, however, as domestic science completed the transition to home economics, the clamor for reform that had characterized the movement for so long began quieting down, and by the 1920s the zealous exertions of the past had relaxed into a pleasant willingness to serve. The turning point came with World War I, for wartime shortages made home economics, especially its nutrition component, an important part of the war effort. With its new relevance home economics was able to make a spectacular surge to legitimacy and emerge from the war effort as a nationally recognized profession. "It nearly killed us off," remarked Isabel Bevier, recalling the hectic demands of those years, "but it made us and our cause eminently respectable."

More firmly established, more securely funded, and more widely accepted than domestic science had ever been, home economics stopped generating leaders or even notable personalities after the war and simply clung to its new status. For all its respectability, however, it was becoming a curiously abstracted career. Despite the scientific research that went on in its graduate schools, despite the meetings devoted to curriculum development, despite the scholarly journals, what kept home economics alive was not its content but its sex. In truth, nothing that went on under the rubric of home economics, whether on campus or in the business world, was unique to the profession: from the study of chemistry and biology to the promotion of new kitchen products, all the work that home economists called their own would have fit nicely under such titles as scientist, or laboratory assistant, or nutritionist, or product tester, or publicist. By calling themselves home economists instead, women created a special, female version of those careers and simply shored up the barriers between what was perceived as women's work and the real world. Women were just beginning to shoulder their way into the professions during the 1920s, but the existence of home economics helped keep the male world male. The few and intensely single-minded females who managed to obtain traditional doctorates in chemistry or biology, for example, found themselves effectively barred from teaching anywhere in a university except the home-economics department. Home economics was the substitute profession for women, a fragile imitation of the larger world rendered in their own terms and limited most drastically by their own pale ambitions. Complacent on their bit of turf, home economists had nothing to professionalize except the role of junior partner to men; under the shelter of a shamelessly irrelevant academic ghetto they contented themselves with producing administrators and functionaries and wives.

Home economics was not the only female profession to blossom after World War I—teaching, nursing, and social work carried greater numbers of women into professional life—but these were identified as women's careers in part because they called upon the best of the qualities traditionally understood as feminine: generosity, selflessness, psychological astuteness. Of course the growth of these professions also depended upon a more evanescent quality of womanhood—the apparent desire to live on ridiculously low pay—but if these women were making a contribution to American life immensely larger than their reward, at least the contribution itself was tangible. Home economics, on the other hand, drew on the most deadening version of femininity available, for the essence of the profession was acquiescence, not action. Working in the kitchens of the food industry to develop new ways of using corn syrup or canned ham, working on the "women's page" of the newspaper or in the household section of a women's magazine, and of course teaching in grade school, high school, and college, the job of a home economist was to manipulate the givens and come up with a set of answers that she knew very well beforehand. The domestic-science movement was hardly famous for its demands on the establishment—indeed, when Mrs. Richards and her colleagues put their faith so wholly in the institutions of industry, commerce, and education, they surrendered their ability to think for themselves—but female servility was never their goal. Yet the most straightforward advice offered by the author of a 1938 text called *Business Opportunities for the Home Economist* was that aspiring careerists in the field cultivate defeat. Writing in the midst of the Depression, the author warned that, with jobs so scarce, women should expect to find businessmen openly prejudiced against female applicants. Even in home economics, where they would not be competing against men, women had no real advantage, for, as the author pointed out, "there is evidence all along the line of a tendency to reduce their status, curtail their authority, and cut their pay." How could women handle this problem? The author passed along some wisdom from an experienced businesswoman: " 'They can read history and accept the fact that they will probably never reach the topmost positions or the highest rewards; they can put aside jealousy and a sense of injustice as profitless and impractical. It would be just as well for students to be taught to lay aside their ambitions for personal glory . . . and to concentrate on doing a worthwhile job even if others get the credit.' "

Women who were able to digest this advice moved into safe positions in the business world, where they were not likely to ask embarrassing questions about the real benefits of the products they were promoting. The supervisor of the American Maize-Products Kitchen, birthplace of Amaizo packaged foods, displayed the right attitude when she enthusiastically described her work for the readers of *American Kitchen* in 1946. "Our basic products are manufactured from corn as the term 'Maize' in our nomen implies," she explained; hence the task of the women working in the experimental kitchen was to dream up "specialized packaged items" using cornstarch, corn oil, and corn syrup. This was not a job for cooks, she noted, but for trained laboratory technicians, and she took her readers step by step through the process of creating a new pudding, tinted yellow but of unnamed flavor. The themes she stressed—the achievement of high standards of quality, uniform results in every package, and foolproof methods of preparation at home—were not very different from the goals of the New England Kitchen. But unlike Mrs. Richards and Mrs. Abel, the Amaizo team had no particular vision of nutritional or moral splendor to guide them. A yellow pudding was its own reward: chief among its virtues, as the author made plain, was that it would be "quite different from anything now appearing on the grocers' shelves." In a similar spirit of achievement, *Better Food Magazine*, a later incarnation of *American Kitchen*, hailed the introduction of the "snow white potato chip," in which manufacturers had managed to eliminate the "objectionable brown color" by passing the potato through still another stage of processing.

The housewife who would greet a new pudding or potato chip with anything like the excitement of its manufacturers had to be virtually manufactured herself, for she certainly had never been born. Beginning in the 1920s, a new image of the American housewife took shape, an image suitable for a new age of material invention and consumption. The advertising industry, the manufacturers of household goods, the food companies, the women's magazines, and the schools all shared in the task of creating a woman who could discriminate among canned soups but who wouldn't ask too many questions about the ingredients: neither angel nor scientist, but homemaker. Unlike "Sally" or "Molly Bishop," those industrious heroines who starred in domestic fiction at the turn of the century and secured both love and social status by learning to cook meals of the proper weight and color, the women who set up housekeeping after World War I were not expected to realize their identities at the kitchen stove.

Between World War I and the Depression the day-to-day work involved in cooking and cleaning changed more dramatically than it would again for another half century. The installation of indoor plumbing and electricity made the biggest difference—these were common by the end of the 1920s—and electric irons, vacuum cleaners, and washing machines were the first of the new appliances to be widely purchased. Wood and coal stoves gave way to gas and electric ranges, and although automatic refrigerators were found only in wealthier households until the mid-1930s, the use of canned and packaged foods was growing steadily. It still took much of a woman's time to keep house, but the hard-labor aspects of the work had lightened and its prominence in the popular image of domesticity was fading. Instead of reveling in daylong meal plans and exhaustive analyses of each cleaning process, as the domestic scientists were fond of doing, experts of this era tended to present the physical work of domesticity as simple necessity, to be executed with speed and skill and all the new appliances, and then sent to the back of one's mind. Heroines of domestic fiction still acknowledged, with their predecessors, that the home was their job just as the office was their husband's, but the job description for women had changed. "Homemaking" involved a great many intangibles that "housekeeping" had only touched on, including the practically limitless role of wife.

In "Love Flies Out of the Kitchen," which ran in the *Ladies' Home Journal* in 1933, a heroine who approaches her domestic role the way Sally and Molly did several decades earlier gets into deep trouble. Lilian is a young wife and mother who one day tells her husband, Steve, that they could economize by firing Dagmar, their servant; Lilian will do all the cooking and housework herself. But this is not a story about the difficulties of learning to cook and clean—on the contrary, the work presents no special problem for Lilian, and at dinner on the first evening of the experiment she sits down in a pretty dress feeling "curiously happy and provocative." This hint of a "provocative" Lilian introduces quite a new element in domestic fiction, and Lilian goes on to make the point outright. " 'Who says that a woman has to choose between being the domestic and the courtesan type?' she inquired of Steve. 'Why should she?' " Her own effort to combine the domestic and the courtesan in a single perfect wife is successful at first, but as the days wear on she finds it more and more of a strain. Soon she begins to neglect the pretty dress and the nicely arranged table and just concentrates on getting her work done. When her husband urges her to come for a drive one evening, she refuses; she has too much to do. As for feeling provocative, she's much too worn out—"deadly tired of just being a cook and housekeeper"—and in a perpetually snappish mood. The only times she feels happy and feminine anymore are the afternoons she spends with Michael, a man she meets at a party, who stops by to visit her often. Michael never finds her anything but charming, for she takes the time to dress up for him, and they have a delightful flirtation, so delightful that Lilian begins to consider leaving her husband. "Was divorce so inconceivable? Shouldn't a woman live, after all, with a man who understood her?" One afternoon, however, he arrives earlier than she expected. Lilian is still wearing the ugly old smock she threw on to serve her husband breakfast, her hair is a mess, and she is screaming at her young son for accidentally spilling a bowl of mayonnaise. Michael's horrified reaction makes it obvious that this visit is his last. Lilian runs to her room in hysterical tears, and that evening she and her husband decide they must rehire Dagmar. " 'I'll go on keeping this house,' " Lilian vows, but now she knows what "keeping house" really means. " 'I'll make a home of it too. I've been doing Dagmar's work, not my own. That's why it's been so hard. I've neglected my job.' "

In this atmosphere the old scientific splendor inherent in household tasks, the intellectual fascination that Ellen Richards was able to perceive in the act of peeling potatoes, became so much flotsam. The nineteenth-century housekeeper—what Lilian would have called the "domestic" type—had very little in common with the twentieth-century homemaker, or "courtesan" type, at least once the house was clean and the family fed. In the world of the homemaker, as manufacturers and retailers hoped to define it, the rigorous analytical attitude that domestic scientists longed to instill in housewives had no place at all. When a group of ambitious homemakers belonging to the District of Columbia Home Economics Association tried to set up a kind of information bank in 1932, recording all the specifics they could obtain as to the quality and construction of various household purchases so that they might make these facts available to other members, they found that the household-goods industry was cold to their inquiries. Talking with store clerks, writing to government research institutes, and trying to learn what lay behind the "seal of approval" bestowed by magazines brought the investigators to the conclusion that industry was not prepared to divulge anything but its ignorance and bias. "The results of our two years' efforts are mostly negative," a member admitted in the *Journal of Home Economics*. The same issue carried an article that perhaps inadvertently explained why. This was a report praising the ways in which the canning industry provided helpful information to consumers. The author was most enthusiastic about a 1931–2 national advertising campaign in which the industry ran newspaper ads for canned foods available in local markets, with "material of general interest concerning canned foods" running in the ostensibly editorial space adjoining the ads. "Such advertising helps to lay the ground work for intelligent buying," concluded the author, who happened to be the home-economics director of the National Canners Association.

Intelligent buying—meaning, of course, the homemaker's willingness to believe what a manufacturer chose to tell her—easily became a more important domestic function than intelligent cooking and cleaning. Home economists working in every sphere seemed to drop the burden of intellectual housekeeping with some relief. Housework was never going to be fun, or even very interesting, and the novelty of fighting germs and disease at home by scrubbing the cellar had long since disappeared. One of the chief differences between housekeeping and homemaking was that, in the course of the latter, women were free to acknowledge that drudgery was drudgery. " 'I don't like housework!' " was the banner announcement on a full-page ad for Bon Ami in 1938. A smiling woman identified as "Mrs. Beach, of Montclair, N.J.," continued, " 'I like Bon Ami for the kitchen sink . . . because I can clean the rest of the kitchen with it at the same time. With a very few extra motions the stove is shining. . . .' " Efficiency, rather than moral superiority, came to be the notable value in cooking and cleaning, and home economists began to direct at least part of their advice to women who hated housework. This was deemed a perfectly acceptable attitude so long as it didn't interfere with one's housework. "Lack of the faculty for success in homemaking, while biologically abnormal, is no disgrace," declared a text by a home-economics professor at Boston University. ". . . It is necessary, however, to make sure that ineptitude is genuine and not a casuist's excuse for the evasion of hard problems and permanent responsibilities." Every homemaker, pointed out another sympathetic expert, "is thrown into her job without regard to its appeal to her. It is a concomitant of marriage. She can not abandon it for another, no matter how difficult she finds it, nor how it bores her."

Once housework had been recognized as neither a science nor a mission, but simply an unalterable element of woman's fate, other aspects of domesticity ballooned. Few home economists were so rash as to suggest, with a Wisconsin teacher, that the best avocation for modern homemakers was more homemaking—by doing extra cooking and sewing, she felt, women would restore to home life "something of its old spirit of adventure and creation" —but the possibilities for a life beyond housework were reduced almost as glibly to the "courtesan type," or perfect wifeliness. In 1953 the *Ladies' Home Journal* began its famous feature "Can This Marriage Be Saved?", a series whose dominant message was made clear early on by the caption under a photograph of a couple embracing in anguish: "Amy was largely responsible for Joe's infidelity. She never took time to be a wife." Standard domestic skills were only a secondary component of wifeliness, which was a service occupation calling for the competence and cajolery of a Mata Hari. " 'I hear so much talk nowadays about being typically feminine," a young woman queried the *Journal*'s Beauty Editor. " 'How does one go about being this way? I always feel so uncomfortable when I try to act "womanly." ' " No wonder. The Beauty Editor responded by describing a "deliciously feminine" woman of her acquaintance, who doesn't talk too much, doesn't laugh too much, is "good company" and "warmly responsive" and "looks as though she would be pleasant to touch." Femininity, in other words, was largely a matter of repression: responding rather than initiating, and acquiescing rather than standing apart. The women who went into factory work during World War II were urged to develop new interests very cautiously as the months and years passed, and not to take up any hobbies or amusements unless they were sure their boyfriends and husbands would want to share them. Education was especially risky, for it might alter the family hierarchy in the wrong direction. Even *Woman's Day*, a magazine distributed through grocery stores and devoted almost entirely to the household, began publication in 1937 with an early feature by Dale Carnegie called "Who's Boss in Your Home?" When your husband comes home and kicks off his dirty overshoes onto the white rug you've just washed, Carnegie asked his readers, how do you react?

His own advice was to swallow any impulse to communicate authentic dismay, and instead to snuggle up and say, " 'My difficult darling, I shall have to wash that rug again today. I mind, really, because I would rather do something to make myself more interesting to you.' "

By the 1950s this image of a wholly compliant femininity, an image shored up equally by commerce and psychology, was rampant. Just as the authors of religious tracts had identified true worthiness in women with domestic self-sacrifice a hundred years earlier, more or less Freudian psychiatrists were now able to guide women toward appropriate fulfillment by reminding them of the joy of subservient home life. Women with other ambitions were increasingly prominent, but these were supposed to be malcontents who personified a garish warning. "You all know women who lack warmth, tenderness, delicacy, and sweetness . . ." one psychiatrist advised a New York lecture audience. "They do not want to be homemakers, they do not want to be mothers. They want to become presiding judges of the Supreme Court. . . ." Such women could suffer "total sexual frigidity, or homosexuality," he cautioned, and even worse than that, this psychosis could result in a woman "separating herself from all that is considered womanly, such as cooking, making a home . . ."

Femininity took on different costumes over the decades—in the Depression years the covers of the *Ladies' Home Journal* showed glamorous women in evening gowns; during World War II, they became defenders of the home front, often in uniform and proudly saluting; and in the 1950s they were cheerful, wholesome wives-and-mothers, typically seen hanging up the wash—but while styles changed and changed again, none of them edged women any closer to autonomy or self-definition. On the contrary, even food advertising stopped appealing to women's sense of themselves—"Dainty Desserts for Dainty People," as the Knox Gelatine Company liked to say—and aimed instead at their sense of duty. " 'I'll be there!' " exclaims a woman on the telephone, in a 1942 Campell's soup ad.

Simultaneously she's responding to her husband ("'I got two tickets for the ball game, dear. How about it?'"), her child ("'Mommy, will you take Doris and me swimming?'"), and a woman in uniform ("'Mrs. Ward, can you be here at the central office for duty at three o'clock?'"). Mrs. Ward's confident attitude is engendered by Campbell's—"'Family meals don't tie me down when soup is the one hot dish!'"—and it's cookery, not family or community responsibility, that is plainly identified as the nuisance here.

Cookery, in fact, went into retreat as the rule of femininity grew more powerful in women's lives. The act of eating, not to mention its indelicate companion, appetite, had long been anathema to femininity, and the reigning value in the modern kitchen was convenience, not coziness, or even apple pie. In one sense, all the elements of scientific cookery triumphed in 1953 with the appearance of the first TV dinner. The subordination of taste and texture, the emphasis on appearance, the flavors that were blunt or nonexistent, and the persistent dream of a nutritional democracy with all Americans eating and flourishing the same way—these standards came to life as boldly as they ever would when the first factory-cut slices of dry white turkey were wrapped around an acrid stuffing and frozen solid. If frozen meals did not, like a culinary Nora, slam the kitchen door once and for all, they did realize a change in perspective that had been creeping into focus for decades. Now cookery could be seen, in the light of technology, as a brief and impersonal relation with food. And food itself could be understood as a simple necessity, one that ought to be manipulated and brought under control as quickly and neatly as bodily functions were handled by modern plumbing.

At the same time, however, the reign of convenience wiped out the one article of faith in scientific cookery that deserved public attention. "Learn to cook in five meals!" the *Journal* was encouraging young brides. Nothing could have been farther from the way the domestic scientists had envisioned the process of learning to cook, for despite their fascination with prepared foods and efficient methods, they carried their understanding of the chemistry of the kitchen as a sacred trust. The *Journal*'s exemplary bride was "learning to cook" by putting canned sauces together with frozen vegetables, and making chocolate pudding out of a package. In other words, she was assembling meals, but as the domestic scientists knew very well, the only way to achieve real efficiency in the kitchen was to learn what to expect from basic ingredients and how to combine them purposefully. Scientific cooks had anticipated the era of culinary regimentation but not the intellectual collapse that would accompany it. In the "money-saving menus" that *Woman's Day* began running in every issue, domestic scientists would have recognized a concept they pioneered themselves a half century earlier, but the *Woman's Day* dinners were organized on a very different principle than the meals typically envisioned by Sarah Tyson Rorer over a two-week period. Mrs. Rorer loved the sense of continuity and completion as boiled mutton became a cold lunch, then hash, then curry. And she would insist on rice and tomatoes with the mutton because she could read nutritional harmony in just such a trio. In contrast, the *Woman's Day* menus were so mechanistic they can only be called degrading to the woman in the kitchen. "Cut 2 boxes frozen cod fillets in halves," went a typical direction. "Broil without turning, as directed on the label." The dishes themselves, based as they were on supermarket packaged foods, were crude imitations of real food—canned luncheon meat baked with brown sugar and honey; "Minted Grapefruit" created by mixing after-dinner mints with grapefruit sections; canned spaghetti baked with bologna; processed American cheese with everything. But it was the cook, not the cooking, that would have most dismayed the domestic scientists. If she could learn to cook in five meals, then learning to cook must not be held a very estimable achievement. And since cooking was still the most pressing day-to-day demand in the household, then women were spending their days doing simpleton's work.

In the last two or three decades, Americans may have started to reverse the lemming-like culinary trends of the previous century. Food writers have attributed the current mania for ethnic food, health food, food fads, kitchen equipment, new restaurants, cookbooks, and cooking lessons to a variety of sources, especially the increase in tourist travel to Europe during the 1950s and the immediate popularity of Julia Child as WGBH-TV's "French Chef" in 1962. Almost at the same time there came a widespread and sustained criticism of the American diet, instigated in the 1960s by the health-food counterculture and replenished continually since then by new findings in nutritional research. *Gourmet* magazine, for years a lonely temple to the refined palate, has been joined by *Bon Appétit, Food and Wine,* and *The Cook's Magazine,* and now these publications are available at the supermarket checkout counter with *Family Circle, Woman's Day,* and *TV Guide.* Today a food processor is standard equpiment in the kitchens of even desultory cooks, and although the rage for Christmas-present pasta machines, gelati makers, and espresso machines has faded somewhat, one can find fresh pasta, rich ice cream made without preservatives, and espresso in any decent-sized city or college town. While the element of fad and fashion cannot be discounted—sushi descends as sun-dried tomatoes rise; kiwis enjoy an enormous vogue and suffer an equally enormous disdain—the common denominators of American taste may well have changed permanently. Quiche and spinach salad, for example, zoomed into the spotlight in the early 1970s but survived their passage through both fashion and cliché to become staples in neighborhood restaurants everywhere. People raised on instant coffee and Wonder Bread are brewing Colombian Supremo and making whole-wheat toast in the morning, and croissants can be picked up in a mall almost as easily as doughnuts. Many of these shifts in popular taste are purely lateral, of course: a typical salad bar, with its iceberg lettuce, Jell-O cubes, polyester tomatoes, and thick orange dressing, is just as discouraging to come across as a typical restaurant salad has always been; the availability of croissants is no guarantee that they will be fresh, or buttery, or in fact anything at all like a croissant. Moreover, while there's no question that it's become easier for people who know the difference to find and cook better food nowadays than at any time since the Industrial Revolution, better food doesn't necessarily mean healthier food. Chemical additives have so dangerously degraded the food supply that in the long run the difference between bologna and steak *au poivre* may come down to little more than the price, the taste, and the company.

Like the food experts of the last century, today's enthusiasts are fully convinced they have rescued food from the barbarous prison of the past. Error and ignorance have been vanquished, according to the popular cooks and writers of our time, and Americans stand at last in culinary triumph over their own ignominious history. At last, like Atwater and his investigators, we know everything we need to know about nutrition, whether perfect health seems to rest this week on fiber or calcium or fat or selenium; at last science has given us an ideal food, whether it's a new sugar substitute or a new ice cream made with tofu, or a new version of orange juice. The revelations accorded in the gospel of nouvelle cuisine have won legions of converts who will never look back. If they did they might see Fannie Farmer, whose passion for novelty led her to marshmallows and candied fruit rather than warm liver salad and lemon-flavored fettucini, but whose impact on a generation was no less powerful for that.

But our contemporary food craze shares more than a blinkered culinary outlook with the craze of the last century: both these manias reflect an obsession with class and style at least as driving as their obsession with dinner. In the late nineteenth century an expanding middle class was using food as a way to define itself, not only by imitating the dainty preferences of the rich, but by carefully avoiding the hallmarks of the poor. Pork, brown bread, thick soups, heavy pies—all these were seen as lower-class, or old-fashioned. Hence the country-bred Polly, in Louisa May Alcott's *An Old-Fashioned Girl*, was pressed to eat macaroons for lunch with her fashionable city acquaintances, while the "honest brown" gingersnaps in her pocket crumbled away. Today the national enthusiasm for food and cookery constitutes a more general expression of unashamed hedonism on the part of a middle class that's pleased with itself. Economical buying and menu planning receive a nod in the newspapers now and then, but the publications devoted to food cheerfully assume a moneyed readership. Such homely dishes as apple crisp and chicken pot pie are enjoying a mid-eighties vogue thanks to a sort of gustatory *nostalgie de la boue*, but they're only on the menu in the most self-assuredly chic restaurants. The near-total concentration on upwardly mobile eating has also resulted in a near-total lack of social consciousness on the part of the new culinary movement. In striking distinction from the last century, today's food experts display little interest in the diet of the poor and hungry. Feeding the helpless is seen as a job for those with a professional interest in such things, not for lovers of fine cooking.

Perhaps the chief difference between the food manias of the present and those of the past lies in the role of eating, which today has taken on respectability and even sublimity of a sort that would have astounded any right-thinking American cook of the nineteenth century. As the agreed-upon social restraints that had long pretended to protect Americans from their feelings began to publicly unravel in the 1960s, gustatory pleasure quickly became overt and then fashionable. Now it's no longer a sign of good breeding and high income to hold oneself above appetite and pick disinterestedly at one's food. On the contrary, those without passion at the table may expect to be pitied. (Society-page journalism represents the last remnant of the domestic-science age in this regard; here reporters still describe the guests at Social Register parties as "nibbling" their elaborate meals.) The use of recipes as a barrier to the senses has been outmoded as well. A confident ability to assemble great meals without showing dependence on cookbooks—the kind of inborn facility that scientific cooks so heartily mistrusted—is now a mark of distinction, indicating as it does that the cook is sensitive to all the vivid smells and flavors and images that awaken appetite. Enthusiastic eating is even more socially appropriate than dieting, although one is certainly not supposed to look fat, gluttonous, or otherwise out of control.

Not surprisingly, the new propriety in eating for pleasure has been slow to take effect in the lives of women. Now, as a hundred years ago, there is something unsettling, something very dimly fearsome, about the sight of a woman putting food of any substantial bulk into her own mouth. What Catharine Maria Sedgwick called the "monster appetite" still haunts women. If the response has changed—anorexia and bulimia are a great deal more common today than green-and-white luncheons or butterfly teas—the apparition has not. Back in 1903 Marion Harland observed that lunch was of no interest to a normal woman, and that since men were tending not to come home in the middle of the day any longer, the middle meal might have disappeared entirely were it not for hungry children. The fiction that women had no appetite for food became a peculiar sort of reality in the 1950s, when dieting seized the public's consciousness: at last it was almost possible to believe that women had no right to food. All the passion and imagination that domestic scientists had devoted to taming the appetite was revived and magnified in the dieting industry. The techniques of cooking had been quietly disappearing on their own, as after-dinner mints teamed up successfully with grapefruit. Now, in place of kitchen wisdom, an infinitude of detail about calorie counting, cottage cheese, and carrot sticks poured out of books and magazines, becoming the center of American culinary life. This gigantic social and commercial enterprise is still with us, and although men now diet chiefly for their health, women continue to diet in homage to a moral asceticism rooted centuries deep.

Mary E. Wilkins Freeman, who wrote a number of spare, gentle stories about village domestic life at the turn of the century, perfectly captured a quintessentially female dinner in her tale "A New England Nun," which describes an evening in the life of Louisa. Having waited for her fiancé through a separation lasting many years, Louisa finds that she's too tenderly attached to all the furnishings of her quiet life alone—the peaceful afternoons sewing a linen seam for the pleasure of it, the bureau drawers fragrant with lavender and clover, the sparkling windowpanes and the tidy rooms that never knew disorder—to want to marry him any longer. One evening, shortly before she decides to tell him so, she arranges her usual solitary supper: ". . . a glass dish full of sugared currants, a plate of little cakes, and one of light white biscuits. Also a leaf or two of lettuce, which she cut up daintily. Louisa was very fond of lettuce, which she raised to perfection in her little garden. She ate quite heartily, though in a delicate, pecking way; it seemed almost surprising that any considerable bulk of the food should vanish." To eat heartily, yet seem to eat nothing; to fill up on lettuce leaves—such a combination of the physical and the discreet, the pleasurable and the insubstantial, smooths over the conflict inherent in femininity and reflects its perfect resolution, the voluptuary of innocence. In our time the symbol of a femininity surpassing the feminine, a more with-it Louisa, might be a model or a ballet dancer: those paper-thin women whose real bodies are sexless, almost shapeless, but whose transmuted image shows a womanhood far more resplendent than life.

Very little in the current food mania is directed at women, and unlike the nineteenth century's craze for cooking, this one does not have women as the leading participants. Women are expected to cook, of course, but in much the same way as they always have—skillfully, automatically, and as close to invisibly as is practicable. Hence advertisements for convenience foods are still aimed at women, but the publicity emanating from the cooking craze is focused on men and couples, those members of society with disposable incomes and a commercial image worth trumpeting. Women on their own, making independent decisions about food they will actually eat rather than serve to others, do not constitute a very appealing class, according to our hardiest prejudices. In recent years women have been moving into the realm of professional cooking in significant numbers, but at its highest levels the world of great cookery is probably more staunchly masculine than the armed forces. Not all male cooks are renowned chefs, of course. Domestic cookery seemed to cross sex lines right around the time sex did, and nowadays there are men who, in traditionally female fashion, prepare ordinary meals for ordinary mealtimes. For the most part, however, women's cooking remains an anonymous service to their families, while men's cooking tends to become a highly personal gift to a grateful audience.

A hundred years ago the women who thought most about food, who talked about it and wrote about it and enshrined it at the head of what they hoped would be a worldwide social and moral revolution, did so to gain control over an appetite they disliked, an appetite that seemed to be peculiarly female. Yet they clung to a notion of femaleness that would undermine the very power they sought. It wasn't the content of the scientific-cookery movement that distinguished it most sharply from feminism, for the suffragists, too, believed that by taking housework seriously they might raise its respectability in the public estimation. What finally relegated domestic scientists to powerless obscurity was their inability to believe in women. For all their inexhaustible study of the subject, they almost never thought to separate woman from woman's work: to them, cooking and housework were sex-linked commitments as definitive as childbearing. And this perspective contented them. They had no wish to deny women the opportunities enjoyed by the most successful domestic scientists—independence, income, travel, a satisfying career—but they had little taste for autonomy. They liked to think of women reaching every star, but only on the female side of the heavens; they liked to think of women as the shadows of men, re-enacting their successes and triumphs, but on the female side of the world. Feminism, as they saw it, had been useful enough in eradicating many of the social and economic disabilities that went with womanhood. Now equality reigned in peace, and woman's new and grave responsibility was to make herself worthy of that equality. What the domestic scientists really believed in was man, and what they wanted for women was progress in his name.

When the Woman's Education Association began supporting a women's chemistry laboratory at MIT in 1876, the rationale at first went no deeper than the title of Ellen Richards's course, "The Chemistry of Cooking and Cleaning." But eight years later, when the laboratory was absorbed into MIT and the doors of the institute proper began opening to women—largely because the association had used its fund-raising ability as leverage in the cause —the members were reflecting on the work of the laboratory in a different, more expansive way. Here, noted the annual report, were young women graduates who could analyze olive oil, vinegar, and baking powder with confidence, who could identify the manufacturers and pinpoint the dealers doing business in such products east of the Mississippi. Here, in short, was a "source of power the extent of which is not yet realized." Not mere acquiescence but power would motivate the domestic lives of these women, the power inherent in a critical knowledge of food manufacturing and distribution. It didn't happen, of course; the food industry has reigned comfortably from that day to this. But for all the narrowness of their vision, the members of the WEA were trying to imagine a feminist future, one in which power and autonomy became decent feminine accomplishments. At the same time, however, Ellen Richards, who had had to cajole her way through the institute as its first female student, went on to oppose the admission of women into MIT on an equal basis with men. As her biographer understood it, Mrs. Richards feared that of the multitudes of women who could be expected to enter the school, only a few would have the brains and stamina to finish, and that such a disparity would strengthen the arguments of those who fought against higher education for women.

At the heart of this reasoning lay the profound mistrust of women that kept Mrs. Richards's words and actions in dizzying contradiction throughout her career. What stopped her short, and blinded the domestic-science movement, was the fear of significant power for women, even that power over themselves "the extent of which is not yet realized." Hence they deployed their ambition in a forum strictly enclosed, their hopes manifestly directed to the male realm outside but their activity securely bound. Like Louisa, who salvaged her independence but lost the chance to share it, these women chose what best reassured them and called it the world. "If Louisa Ellis had sold her birthright she did not know it, the taste of the pottage was so delicious, and had been her sole satisfaction for so long," the story concludes. "She gazed ahead through a long reach of future days strung together like pearls in a rosary, every one like the others, and all smooth and flawless and innocent, and her heart went up in thankfulness." Smooth and flawless and innocent—a life as perfect as a molded salad inspired the domestic scientists, and they never dreamed of wanting food.

Acknowledgments

Convention dictates that one's husband be thanked last, but in the case of so unusual a husband as Jack Hawley, convention fails. His early and persistent faith in this project, as well as a presumably unfeigned interest in the minutiae of domestic science, have made him the first cornerstone.

Gratitude of another sort goes to the National Endowment for the Humanities, which supported my work with a Fellowship for Independent Study and Research, and to Les Dames d'Escoffier for a grant enabling me to make use of the extraordinary culinary collection at the Schlesinger Library.

Many friends put their minds to this project at one stage or another, and for their ideas, advice, and encouragement I'm grateful to Joyce Antler, Dorothy Austin, Joe Carlin, Lois Edgerly, Tom Friedman, Dolores Hayden, Tom Lam, Steve Monk, Gail Parker, Susan Pelzer, Adele Pressman, Paul Solman, Susie Strasser, Suzanne Weil, Gwen Wright, and the members of my Cambridge writers' group: Ann Banks, Celia Gilbert, Janet Murray, Beth O'Sullivan, Harriet Reisen, Claire Rosenfield, Marjorie Shostak, and Barbara Sirota. Henry Deeks started me off on my research by alerting me to a stash of Fannie Farmer memorabilia gleaned from the remnants of Miss Farmer's School of Cookery. The chapter on Fannie Farmer owes a great deal to Margo Miller, who saved me months of work by generously sharing the results of her own extensive research. The family of Lucy Allen gave me access to many of Miss Allen's cooking-school papers and allowed me to keep some of the treasures I found, and Marion Atwood was entertaining and enlightening on the culinary career of her sister Alice Bradley. To Barbara Wheaton I owe the discovery, at a shockingly late date, that my book was trying to define what made American cooking American.

From the beginning, John Sterling and Jonathan Galassi supported my tenuous plans with enthusiasm that remained a source of comfort as the years dragged by. Brenda Peterson's insights and brainstorms made an immeasurable contribution to this book and many times gave me the courage to type. And the kind, brainy guidance of my agent, Amanda Urban, and my editor, Pat Strachan, have made me feel like the most richly blessed writer in the world, even at those times when all evidence went firmly to the contrary.

Finally, and with a deep, heartfelt curtsy, I must acknowledge that this book, like so many others, would not have been possible without the manifold resources of the Schlesinger Library and the jewel in its crown, Barbara Haber.

L.S.

Notes

Prologue

3. "Q: Are Vegetables ever served": *American Cookery*, June–July 1923, p. 53.

5. "Looking at the affairs": Maude Hanson Lacy, "Woman's Point of View; Its Effect Upon the Home," *New England Kitchen Magazine*, April 1898, p. 7. *New England Kitchen Magazine* began publication in April 1894, changed its name to *American Kitchen Magazine* with the issue of September 1898, and later was published under the names *Home Science, Modern Housekeeping*, and *Everyday Housekeeping.*

One

11. "domestic saints": Harriet Beecher Stowe, "The Cathedral." Quoted in Gail Parker, ed., *The Oven Birds*, p. 205.

11. best-selling novelist: See Elizabeth Stuart Phelps, below.

12. "A servant by this clause": from "The Elixir," by George Herbert. The poem, beginning "Teach me, my God and King," was published in 1633 and set to its familiar tune by William Crotch in 1836. See, for example, Marion Harland's "Familiar Talk with My Fellow-Housekeeper and Reader" in her manual *Common Sense in the Household* (1871): "My dear, John and the children, and the humble home, make your sphere for the present, you say. Be sure you fill it—*full!* before you seek one wider and higher. There is no better receipt between these covers than that. Leave the rest to GOD. Everybody knows those four lines of George Herbert's which ought to be framed and hung up in the work-room of every house . . ." (p. 20).

12. the early 1800s: See Nancy F. Cott, *The Bonds of Womanhood*; Susan Strasser, *Never Done*; and Ann Douglas, *The Feminization of American Culture* for discussion and analyses of American women and domesticity in the eighteenth and nineteenth centuries.

15. widely read poetry: e.g., "Cuthbert," by Susie M. Best (*Table Talk*, June 1892, p. 223) and "The Sweeper of the Floor," by George MacDonald (*New England Kitchen Magazine*, April 1898, p. 9).

16. "Few persons, probably": Catharine M. Sedgwick, *Home*, p. 13.

17. "image of heaven": *Ibid.*, p. 13.

17. "a loving and": *Ibid.*, p. 11.

17. "tawdry pictures": *Ibid.*, p. 18.

17. "There was a disinfecting principle": *Ibid.*, pp. 20–1.

17. "*three lessons*": *Ibid.*, p. 28.
17. a few strawberries: *Ibid.*, p. 31.
17. "The monster appetite": *Ibid.*, p. 33.
18. "can't be expected": *Ibid.*, pp. 42–3.
18. "The Reverse of the Picture": *Ibid.*, p. 44.
18. " 'it has quite a home look' ": *Ibid.*, p. 139.
18. " 'spirit of cultivation' ": *Ibid.*, p. 141.
18. "Death has no sting": *Ibid.*, p. 158.
19. the divorce rate: Carl Degler, *At Odds*, pp. 166–9.
19. edge of bitterness: For another view of Phelps, see Ann Douglas, *The Feminization of American Culture.*
20. "It was impossible": Elizabeth Stuart Phelps, *The Story of Avis*, p. 283.
20. "cold, smooth theorizing": Phelps, *The Gates Ajar*, p. 109.
20. an angel: Phelps, *Chapters from a Life*, p. 95. ("The angel said unto me 'Write!' and I wrote.")
20. " 'some mountains' " Phelps, *The Gates Ajar*, p. 137.
20. " ' "preparing" my home' ": *Ibid.*, p. 139.
20. " 'What could be done' ": *Ibid.*, p. 140.
21. " 'P'r'aps I'll have' ": *Ibid.*, p. 183.
21. " 'I don't see how' ": *Ibid.*, p. 181.
21. "A certain indefinable": *Ibid.*, p. 223.
22. "The old ache": Phelps, *Beyond the Gates*, p. 187.
23. "It is all unfamiliar": Phelps, *The Gates Between*, p. 153.
23. "Here in this world": *Ibid.*, p. 178.
23. "I wished to": *Ibid.*, p. 214.
24. " '. . . these little trials' ": Sedgwick, *Married or Single?* Vol. II, p. 47.
24. "With more of such": *Idem.*
26. Born in 1800: See Kathryn Kish Sklar, *Catharine Beecher: A Study in American Domesticity.*
29. "Supreme Lawgiver": Catharine Beecher, *A Treatise on Domestic Economy*, p. 2.
29. "it is decided that": *Ibid.*, p. 4.
29. "that a few may live": *Idem.*
29. "already the light": *Ibid.*, p. 12.
29. "The proper education": *Ibid.*, p. 13.
29. "refined and lady-like": *Ibid.*, p. 39.
29. "drudgery" and "dirty work": *Ibid.*, p. 40.
29. "It is because": *Idem.*
30. "It may, at first": *Ibid.*, p. 434.
30. "the most important": *Ibid.*, p. 144.
31. "appointed by Perfect Wisdom": *Ibid.*, p. 141.
31. "habits of system": *Ibid.*, p. 142.
31. "persons of moderate circumstances": *Ibid.*, p. 275.
31. "most of the domestic": *Ibid.*, p. 282.
31. "the most soiling employments": *Idem.*

32. the "Christian family": Catharine Beecher and Harriet Beecher Stowe, *The American Woman's Home*, p. 455.

32. the "highest kind": *Ibid.*, p. 457.

Two

34. " 'I have been keeping' ": Christine Frederick papers. Mrs. Frederick typed up a list of the queries she had received from April to September 1913, heading them "How Can I Run My Home More Easily."

35. "Is it not pitiful": Mrs. M. V. Shailer, "The Practical Solution of the Domestic Service Problem," *New England Kitchen Magazine*, February 1898, p. 177.

35. "Suppose my cellar": F. H. Rowley, "Clean Homes," *Good Housekeeping*, May 30, 1885, p. 13.

36. " 'You were in' ": Evelyn M. Wood-Lovejoy, "Left-Handed Housekeeping," *American Kitchen Magazine*, November 1901, pp. 63–4.

36. The "ideal housekeeper": Catherine Owen, *Progressive Housekeeping*, pp. 7–8.

37. "A man must": Emma P. Ewing, "The Untrained Hand," *Boston Cooking-School Magazine*, June–July 1899, p. 2.

37. A Vassar graduate: See Caroline Hunt, *The Life of Ellen H. Richards*; Roberta Frankfort, *Collegiate Women*, pp. 104–10; and Robert Clarke, *Ellen Swallow*.

38. a "Radical": Hunt, p. 91.

38. " 'new and wider' ": *Ibid.*, p. 142.

38. Household Chemistry: Woman's Education Association Annual Report, 1878, p. 7.

39. the "center for": Clarke, p. 69.

39. "Woman was originally": Ellen H. Richards, "Domestic Science: What it is and How to Study it at Home," *The Outlook*, April 24, 1897, p. 1079.

40. "help the housewife": *Idem.*

40. "Was she beguiled": Richards, "The Place of Science in Woman's Education," *New England Kitchen Magazine*, September 1897, p. 226. (This was an address delivered at the dedication of Science Hall, Lake Erie Seminary, Painesville, Ohio.)

40. a "long step": Richards, "Housekeeping in the Twentieth Century," *American Kitchen Magazine*, March 1900, p. 203.

41. "We need to exalt": *New England Kitchen Magazine*, July 1897, p. 167.

41. "If the piano": *American Kitchen Magazine*, March 1900, p. 221. The unnamed weekly paper may have been quoting Mrs. Margaret Sangster, author of *Winsome Womanhood*, among many other works, who once stated, "There is nothing occult or difficult about housework. I do not think there is anything about it a woman

could not learn in six weeks and learn much better in a home than she could in a training school." (Quoted in *Good Housekeeping*, October 1897, p. 162.)

42. "The daily treadmill": Hanna Otis Brun, "Household Inventions," *New England Kitchen Magazine*, January 1896, p. 157.

42. "The woman who": Richards, "The Relation of College Women to Progress in Domestic Science," paper presented to the Association of Collegiate Alumnae on October 24, 1890.

42. "From lowly tasks": Irma T. Jones, "Ethics of the Kitchen," *New England Kitchen Magazine*, November 1894, p. 112.

43. "Would not such": Anna Barrows, "The Apple in Cookery," *New England Kitchen Magazine*, October 1894, p. 30.

43. "that she was a lady": *New England Kitchen Magazine*, December 1894, p. 148.

43. "generally wealthy families": *New England Kitchen Magazine*, March 1898, p. 240.

43. "Washington's daintiest people": "Washington Food Exposition," *Household News*, March 1894, p. 344.

44. "a dainty dish": Sarah Tyson Rorer, "Our Bills of Fare," *Household News*, April 1894, pp. 384–6. "A new culinary adjective is to be desired," *American Kitchen Magazine* finally admitted. "Dainty, attractive and the like are much overworked, but we are not sure that a western newspaper has made any distinct advance when it tells us of a 'dressy soup' " (January 1900, p. 160).

44. "Twenty years ago": Hunt, p. 286.

44. "Woman—with a capital letter": Quoted in Lydia Hoyt Farmer, ed., "Domestic Science in American Homes," *What America Owes to Women*, Charles Wells Moulton, 1893, p. 120.

45. "If I were asked": Quoted in Aileen Kraditor, *Up from the Pedestal*, p. 318.

Three

48. " 'She would reform' ": F. O. Matthiessen, ed., *The American Novels and Short Stories of Henry James*, New York, Knopf, 1947, p. 426.

48. "The wide-spread interest": Woman's Education Association Annual Report, 1880, p. 12.

49. "Cambridge notabilities": Mothers Club of Cambridge club records, March 1885.

50. "Your memory of": James Russell Lowell, quoted in Arthur Bernon Tourtellot, *The Charles*, New York, Farrar and Rinehart, 1941, p. 288–9.

50. "fortified intrenchments": Quoted in "Letter of the Commissioner of Education to the Secretary of the Interior," *Training Schools of Cookery*, p. 7.

50. "There are many": *Ibid.*, p. 6. The commissioner was quoting from a letter written by Harriet N. Noyes, "chairman of the

industrial committee of the Young Woman's Christian Association, Boston."

51. "While this Committee": Woman's Education Association Annual Report, 1874, p. 4.

53. a "competent teacher": Boston Cooking School Committee, Minutes of the Meetings, March 8, 1879.

54. "advertisements and editorials": *Ibid.*, March 5, 1879.

54. "daughters of mechanics": *Ibid.*, February 21, 1879.

54. "should be given": *Ibid.*, March 8, 1879.

54. According to respectful: the *Boston Evening Transcript*, March 10, 1879; the *Boston Advertiser*, March 11, 1879.

56. "who wish to make": Boston Cooking School Committee minutes, March 17, 1879.

56. "to such poor": *Idem.*

56. "should be restricted": *Ibid.*, April 4, 1879.

57. "This gave me": Mary Lincoln, "How I Was Led to Teach Cookery," *New England Kitchen Magazine*, May 1894.

58. "The Committee feel": Woman's Education Association Annual Report, 1881, p. 12.

59. "Henceforth": Boston Cooking School Committee minutes, December 5, 1882.

59. "The attempt to": The Boston Cooking School First Annual Report, 1884, p. 13.

59. "The original purpose": Woman's Education Association Annual Report, 1883, p. 10.

60. a "class of housekeepers": *Ibid.*, p. 11.

60. ". . . that a woman is rich": The Boston Cooking School First Annual Report, 1884, p. 13.

61. "Why does not": *Ibid.*, p. 12.

61. "slower . . . than had": *Ibid.*, p. 1.

61. "has been smaller": *Ibid.*, p. 13.

61. "Cooks will not": Woman's Education Association Annual Report, 1883, p. 11.

62. "a much-to-be-desired": Woman's Education Association Annual Report, 1904, p. 28.

62. The New York school: Juliet Corson, *Cooking School Text Book and Housekeepers' Guide*, pp. 25, 66, 103, 143.

63. In all three courses: "Course of Instruction at the Boston Cooking School" (leaflet).

65. "to lift this": The Boston Cooking School First Annual Report, 1884, p. 10.

65. At the height: Janet McKenzie Hill, "The Boston Cooking-School," *Boston Cooking-School Magazine*, August–September 1898, p. 77.

66. "The demand is": Gertrude Coburn, "Domestic Economy in a College Course," *American Kitchen Magazine*, December 1898, p. 90.

66. The ceremonies honoring: "Commencement of '97 at the Boston Cooking School," *Boston Cooking-School Magazine*, August–September 1897, pp. 92–7. Alice Bradley went on to become a well-known cook and teacher, succeeding Fannie Farmer as principal of Miss Farmer's School of Cookery.

69. In the summer: "News Items and Reports," *New England Kitchen Magazine*, June–July 1894, pp. 174–83.

69. Reports from local: Mrs. Perry, Miss Young, and Mrs. Lincoln, in *New England Kitchen Magazine*, May 1894, pp. 107–8; Miss Clarke and Miss Nichols, in *New England Kitchen Magazine*, June–July 1894, p. 184.

Four

71. "Now, what does": Lincoln, "Extracts from Cookery, or Art and Science versus Drudgery and Luck," in Mary Eagle, ed., *The Congress of Women*, p. 139.

72. "I am afraid": Rorer, "Answers to Inquiries," *Household News*, February 1894, p. 304.

73. " 'I came home' ": Harland, "Martha and Her American Kitchen," *The Woman's Home Companion*, June 1905, p. 7.

75. "We live more intensely": W. O. Atwater, "What We Should Eat," *The Century*, June 1888, p. 259.

76. " 'Let's see—' ": Alice Bradley, "Household Engineering" (clipping from an unidentified newspaper, June 1919; Marietta Greenough papers).

77. Boiled Mutton: Printed copies of the recipes were distributed at the public lecture-demonstrations given at the Boston Cooking School and Miss Farmer's School of Cookery. Many of these demonstration slips survive among the papers of women who attended the lectures or were employed at the schools.

77. According to Atwater: Atwater, Bulletin 21, Office of Experiment Stations, U.S. Department of Agriculture, 1895, p. 73.

77. "Some acid condiment": Lincoln, "From Day to Day," *American Kitchen Magazine*, September 1901, p. 221.

77. As Atwater had shown: Atwater, "The Composition of Our Bodies and Our Food," *The Century*, May 1887, pp. 69, 71. See also Atwater, "The Digestibility of Food," *The Century*, September 1887, p. 736.

78. "an exceedingly wise": Rorer, "Our Bills of Fare," *Household News*, October 1893, p. 114.

78. "Mock Indian Pudding": Fannie Farmer, *The Boston Cooking-School Cook Book*, p. 329.

78. "The reaping of grain": W. T. Sedgwick, "On External Digestion, Commonly Called Alimentation," in *Plain Words About Food*, pp. 45, 47.

79. "a kind of cooking": Lincoln, "Extracts from Cookery," p. 140.

79. "We live upon": Atwater, "The Digestibility of Food," p. 733. He was quoting Meinert.

79. a famous series: See Beecher, *A Treatise on Domestic Economy*, p. 82, and Andrew Combe, *The Physiology of Digestion*, pp. 98–129.

80. "Life," she used to: Rorer, *Mrs. Rorer's New Cook Book*, p. 182.

80. The meal began: Rorer, "Our Bills of Fare," *Household News*, January 1894, p. 259.

80. "Without the appetizing": Richards and Elliott, *The Chemistry of Cooking and Cleaning*, pp. 61, 59.

80. Atwater was less certain: Atwater, "The Digestibility of Food," pp. 739–40.

81. analyzing the digestive function: Lincoln, "From Day to Day," *American Kitchen Magazine*, October 1900, pp. 25–6.

82. "Dishes containing meat": Richards, *Dietary Computer*, p. 14.

82. ROAST STUFFED HEART: *Ibid.*, p. 20.

83. "The recipes are not": *Ibid.*, p. 3.

83. "There is probably": "Everyday Breakfasts," *American Kitchen Magazine*, October 1899, p. 18.

84. Mrs. Lincoln once shared: Lincoln, "From Day to Day," *American Kitchen Magazine*, August 1902, pp. 199–200.

84. a Bulgarian color scheme: "Menus for October Luncheons and Teas," *Boston Cooking School Magazine*, October 1913, p. 185.

84. otherwise thoroughly pink: Rorer, "Housekeepers Inquiries," *Table Talk*, May 1892, p. 170.

84. the all-white meal: See *Table Talk*, May 1892 ("Lily Lunch," p. 170; "White Rose Dinner," p. 174) and June 1892, p. 223, where Mrs. Rorer describes a white dinner flecked with green, planned for the closing exercises of the Philadelphia Cooking School.

85. "Take any kind": "Good Things for the Table," *Good Housekeeping*, May 2, 1885, p. 22.

85. Women wrote constantly: "dried peaches" and "doughnuts" in Lincoln, "From Day to Day," *American Kitchen Magazine*, December 1901, pp. 111–12; "pickling" in Rorer, "Answers to Inquirers," *Household News*, September 1893, p. 86; "corn flour and corn meal," in Rorer, "Answers to Inquirers," *Household News*, November 1893, p. 178; "pie crust," in *Ibid.*, p. 172; and "pound cake" in "Queries and Answers," *Boston Cooking School Magazine*, April 1904, p. 474.

86. "Mrs. Tripp has": Lizzie Goodenough diary, June 29, July 8, August 24, 1865.

86. "even the intelligent": Helen Campbell, *Household Economics*, pp. 16–17. The book is derived from a series of lectures she delivered at the University of Wisconsin in 1895.

86. " 'The only things' ": Mary Wade, "Cooking-School Methods

in Every-Day Life," *New England Kitchen Magazine*, April 1895, p. 14.

87. Traditionally a European: I am indebted to Barbara Wheaton for this perspective.

87. "What I Have for Breakfast": "The Help-One-Another Club," *The Woman's Home Companion*, November 1904, pp. 54–5.

89. "to learn principles": See Lincoln, "From Day to Day," *New England Kitchen Magazine*, October 1895, p. 25. "It is a gratifying and significant fact that but few if any requests have come to us for menus for the entire month. Indeed we have heard many expressions of pleasure that our pages have not been filled with these usually unsatisfactory details." See also *New England Kitchen Magazine*, November 1895, p. 97.

89. "simple, practical": "Menus for April," *New England Kitchen Magazine*, April 1898, p. 28.

89. A suitably quick: *Ibid.*, pp. 28–9.

89. If a massive noon dinner: "Menus for November," *American Kitchen Magazine*, November 1898, p. 70.

90. "The liver terrapin": Rorer, "Our Bills of Fare," *Household News*, July 1893, pp. 3–4.

90. "Housekeeping handed down": Barrows, "Manual Training as a Factor in Home Life," *New England Kitchen Magazine*, October 1895, pp. 5–6.

91. "The savage tears": *The Boston Cooking School Magazine*, August–September 1899, p. 76.

91. the humble carrot: Lincoln, *The Boston Cook Book*, pp. 302–5.

91. Unappetizing winter beets: Margaret Hamilton Welch, "Domestic Topics," *Harper's Bazaar*, January 1904, p. 101.

91. "when they were covered": Barrows, "The Cookery of Milk and Cheese," *New England Kitchen Magazine*, April 1895, p. 23. This was a lecture given before the Maine State Dairy Conference.

91. "Frankfort sausages": Boston Cooking School demonstration slip, February 17, 1897, Marietta Greenough papers.

91. A turkey garnished: "Seasonable Dishes for January," *American Kitchen Magazine*, January 1901, p. 201.

91. pieces of steamed halibut: Lincoln, "From Day to Day," *American Kitchen Magazine*, August 1902, p. 201.

92. sinking a boiled chicken: Rorer, "Corn Kitchen," *Household News*, November 1893, p. 171.

92. August 4, 1899: "New Menus for August," *Table Talk*, August 1899, p. 299.

92. "an ample and satisfactory luncheon": Lincoln, "From Day to Day," *New England Kitchen Magazine*, July 1897, p. 153.

92. a Mormon woman: Mary Ann Hafen in Christiane Fischer, ed., *Let Them Speak for Themselves*, p. 103.

92. Lecturing to a Minnesota audience: Corson, *A Course of*

Lectures on the Principles of Domestic Economy ond Cookery, p. 10.

93. "Often richness or moisture": Hill, "Cookery for Young Housekeepers," *Boston Cooking School Magazine*, March 1908, p. 381.

93. "a dish called": Corson, *A Course of Lectures*, p. 24.

93. a "*chaud-froid*": Rorer, "Mrs. Rorer's Answers to Questions," *Ladies' Home Journal*, March 1897, p. 36.

94. "The secret of": "The Help-One-Another Club," *The Woman's Home Companion*, July 1904, p. 37.

94. Boiled cod, mashed potatoes: Christine Terhune Herrick, "Cottage Dinners," *Ladies' Home Journal*, January 1887, p. 9, and March 1887, p. 9.

94. The kitchen itself: See Gwendolyn Wright, *Moralism and the Model Home*, p. 120.

94. "There should be": "World's Food Fair," *New England Kitchen Magazine*, October 1894, pp. 3–4.

95. "Vegetables are rich": Lincoln, *Mrs. Lincoln's Boston Cook Book*, p. 291.

95. "salts": See Rorer, *Mrs. Rorer's New Cook Book*, p. 10; and Mrs. Bayard Taylor, *Letters to a Young Housekeeper*, p. 98.

95. "Last, but not least": Taylor, p. 98.

95. According to the syllabus: Mary Chambers, "Lessons in the Economics of Nutrition and Practical Cookery," *Boston Cooking School Magazine*, February 1902, pp. 306–7.

96. Most authorities recommended: Lincoln, *Mrs. Lincoln's Boston Cook Book*, p. 298 (string beans); Rorer, *Ladies' Home Journal*, June 1897, p. 25 (asparagus and cucumbers); Welch, *Harper's Bazaar*, January 1904, p. 101 (beets).

96. "ribbons of uniform width": Hill, *Practical Cooking and Serving*, p. 325.

96. a spinach salad: See Harland, *Common Sense in the Household*, p. 225, and Farmer, *The Boston Cooking-School Cook Book*, p. 396.

96. "Arrange the lettuce": Lincoln, "A Winter Dinner," *New England Kitchen Magazine*, February 1895, pp. 251–2.

97. the "downstairs" table: Owen, *Progressive Housekeeping*, p. 129.

97. "Surely no lady": Lincoln, "A Winter Dinner," pp. 251–2.

97. "I never allow": Taylor, p. 150.

98. Squares of frozen: Josephine Grenier, "A Bride's Dinner," *Harper's Bazaar*, June 1904, p. 628 (squares of frozen cream cheese); Mary Foster Snider, "Decorations for a Golf Luncheon," *Table Talk*, October 1902, p. 392 (Golf Salad); unidentified clippings in the Marietta Greenough papers (Salad Mousse, Porcupine Salad, several varieties of Waldorf Salad).

98. "close, firm, solid heads": Barrows and Lincoln, *The Home Science Cook Book*, p. 153.

98. Other popular ways: Boston Cooking School demonstration

slip, February 12, 1902, Marietta Greenough papers (apple-celery-and-mayonnaise salad); Christine Herrick, *The New Idea Home and Cook Book*, p. 103 (banana-and-nut salad); Hill, "Seasonable Recipes," *Boston Cooking School Magazine*, January 1912, p. 287 (marinated peas); Farmer, "My Twelve Favorite Recipes," *The Woman's Home Companion*, April 1905, p. 35 (fruit salad); "A Dinner for Six," *American Kitchen Magazine*, January 1903, p. 144 (red pepper and asparagus); Hill, "Seasonable Recipes," *Boston Cooking School Magazine*, April 1904, p. 461 (string-bean salad); Lincoln, "From Day to Day," *American Kitchen Magazine*, December 1898, p. 135 (frozen celery salad).

99. "Could you give": Henrietta Rowe Morrill, "Winter Salads," *American Kitchen Magazine*, March 1903, p. 233 (cheese salad); Barrows, "Dishes for Midsummer," *American Kitchen Magazine*, July 1902, p. 153 (chicken salad); Lincoln, "From Day to Day," *New England Kitchen Magazine*, May 1896, p. 87 (jellied fruit); Morrill, *op. cit.* (jellied fruit salad).

100. Perfection Salad: According to Jane and Michael Stern, *Square Meals*, p. 139, Perfection Salad first appeared as the third-prize winner in a contest sponsored by Knox Gelatin in 1905. Under the name "Jellied Vegetables" it appeared in the 1906 edition of *The Boston Cooking-School Cook Book*. Knox Gelatin featured the recipe in its booklets for many years.

100. "Edible Flowers": "World's Food Fair," *New England Kitchen Magazine*, October 1894, pp. 9–10.

101. "Foods That Tickle": Demonstration slip, Miss Farmer's School of Cookery, March 20, 1912 (Edith Raymond papers).

101. the "green sickness": See Joan Jacobs Brumberg, "Chlorotic Girls, 1870–1920: A Historical Perspective on Female Adolescence," *Child Development*, 1982, 53, pp. 1468–77.

101. "How to Eat": Margaret Sidney, "How to Eat, Drink, and Sleep as a Christian Should," *Good Housekeeping*, January 9, 1886, p. 126.

102. Commonly recommended: Grenier, "Men's Dinners," *Harper's Bazaar*, March 1904, pp. 305–7.

102. "What Husbands Like": Demonstration slip, Miss Farmer's School of Cookery, March 13, 1912 (Edith Raymond papers).

102. "It is too artistic": Lincoln, "A Lecture on Salads," *New England Kitchen Magazine*, June 1895, p. 131. Report of a lecture given at a meeting of the Massachusetts Household Economic Association.

102. miniature cabbages: Lincoln, "From Day to Day," *New England Kitchen Magazine*, October 1895, pp. 29–30.

103. the fish was molded: Demonstration slip, Boston Cooking School, March 9, 1898 (Marietta Greenough papers).

103. "Kate Douglas Wiggin": "Chafing Dish Cookery," *American Kitchen Magazine*, October 1900, p. 150. The article mentioned

seven chafing-dish cookbooks by popular authorities including Gesine Lemcke, Christine Terhune Herrick, Janet McKenzie Hill, and Fannie Farmer.

103. "We have looked": *American Kitchen Magazine*, April 1900, p. 36.

104. "This lesson shows": Lincoln, "A Lecture on Salads," p. 131.

104–5. an immensely popular serial: Owen, *Ten Dollars Enough*. The serial ran for a year, beginning November 14, 1885, and then was published as a book. Page references are to the book. "Stupid-looking," p. 8; "doing things daintily," p. 14; "penniless Molly," p. 3; " 'You vulgar little person!' " p. 20; "rapid boiling," p. 24; " 'I assure you,' " p. 2.

Five

107. "something which every": "Glad Tidings to the Housekeeper," *The Woman's Home Companion*, August 1905, p. 55.

107. Lamb chops standing: Lincoln, "My Twelve Favorite Recipes," *The Woman's Home Companion*, February 1905, pp. 23, 32.

107. oysters and canned tomatoes: Farmer, "My Twelve Favorite Recipes," *The Woman's Home Companion*, April 1905, pp. 34–5, 49.

108. "notable housewife": Mary Bronson Hartt, "Fannie Merritt Farmer—An Appreciation," *The Woman's Home Companion*, December 1915, p. 21.

108. "these cooking-school messes": Letter from Wilma Lord Perkins to Margo Miller, 1974. Mrs. Perkins was the widow of Dexter Perkins, Miss Farmer's nephew.

108. "Unitarian and bookish": *Ibid.*

109. one apocryphal story: See, for example, the entry on Fannie Farmer in James, *Notable American Women*, Volume 1, p. 597, and "Fannie Farmer's Life Story, One of Magnificent Courage," in the *Boston Herald*, September 8, 1947.

109. She did so well: The various sources on Fannie Farmer's biographical data are contradictory, but according to a typescript of one of her obituaries, she was graduated from the Boston Cooking School in 1889, after completing what would have been a six-month normal course. According to a biographical sketch printed in *The Woman's Home Companion* in 1914—during her tenure at the magazine, that is, and presumably accurate—she followed her graduation with "a year's practical experience as a housekeeper." This probably means that she stayed home until a teaching offer came from the Boston Cooking School in 1891. See "Our Own Folks," *The Woman's Home Companion*, March 1914, p. 1.

110. "the brightest star": Lincoln, "Mrs. Dearborn," *New England Kitchen Magazine*, May 1895, p. 60.

110. "There was little": "The Boston Cooking School," *New England Kitchen Magazine*, April 1894, p. 4.

110. "trying time": *Ibid.*, pp. 4–5.

111. "Miss F. says": Notebook, Lucy Allen papers (collection of the author).

111. "I for one": Farmer, "New Ways of Using Vegetables," *The Woman's Home Companion*, October 1905, p. 44.

111. "Our instructors love": Isabel Gordon Curtis, "A Visit to the Boston Cooking School," *Good Housekeeping*, December 1900, p. 320.

112. liked to eat: Farmer, "The Sweet Course," *The Woman's Home Companion*, February 1911, p. 50. Here Fannie Farmer praises sugar for providing "one of our most delightful flavors."

112. Miss Farmer felt: Wilma Lord Perkins to Margo Miller.

113. "The book is well": "Book Reviews," *New England Kitchen Magazine*, February 1897, pp. 237–8.

113. "All articles to": Lincoln, *Mrs. Lincoln's Boston Cook Book*, p. 15.

114. "Great care must": Farmer, *The Boston Cooking-School Cook Book*, p. 23.

115. "Correct measurements are": *Ibid.*, p. 27.

115. Half-pint measuring cups: See Rorer, *Table Talk*, May 1887, p. 139, quoted in Emma Weigley, *Sarah Tyson Rorer*: "'. . . a small tin kitchen cup that has recently made its appearance in our market. They are sold in pairs at various prices . . . one of the pair is divided into quarters and the other into thirds.'" In 1892 the cups cost twenty cents a pair (Rorer, *Table Talk*, March 1892, p. 108). In 1894 Mrs. Rorer included measuring spoons and measuring cups in a list of essential kitchen furnishings (*Household News*, February 1894, p. 310).

115. "just rounded over": Lincoln, *Mrs. Lincoln's Boston Cook Book*, p. 29.

116. "*A cupful*": Farmer, *The Boston Cooking-School Cook Book*, pp. 27, 28.

116. the "Mother": See Jane Nickerson, "Best-Seller—And Cooks' Friend," *The New York Times Magazine*, October 7, 1945, p. 16.

117. Soon after she became principal: The Boston Cooking School moved to 372 Boylston Street during the winter of 1897–98. For the success of the school under Fannie Farmer, see abstracts of the annual reports published in the *Boston Cooking School Magazine*, February–March 1898, p. 277; April–May 1899, p. 289; February–March 1900, p. 226; February–March 1901, p. 214; and "News and Notes," October 1901, p. 140.

118. began to grow away: See "Our Own Folks," *The Woman's Home Companion*, March 1914, p. 1, and "Boston Cooking Class," *Bulletin of the Inter-Municipal Commitee on Household Research*, March 1905, pp. 10–11.

118. "plain and fancy cooking": "News and Notes," *Boston Cooking School Magazine*, October 1901, p. 140.

118. a drab school year: "News and Notes," *Boston Cooking School Magazine*, August–September 1901, p. 92.

118. the "most prosperous": "News and Notes," *Boston Cooking School Magazine*, June–July 1902, n.p.

119. A few months later: See notice headed "Simmons College Transfer of Boston Cooking School," in *Boston Cooking School Magazine*, March 1904, p. xxvi, and Kenneth L. Mark, *Delayed by Fire*, p. 36.

119. eventually had four kitchens: "Our Own Folks," *The Woman's Home Companion*, March 1914, p. 1; "Boston Cooking Class," *Bulletin of the Inter-Municipal Committee on Household Research*, March 1905, pp. 10–11; and brochure, Miss Farmer's School of Cookery, 1912–13.

120. "I am enclosing": Fannie Farmer to Emma L. Morrow, March 19, 1912 (collection of Margo Miller).

121. When she made croquettes: Farmer, "How to Make Croquettes," *The Woman's Home Companion*, January 1911, p. 43, and Farmer, *A New Book of Cookery*, pp. 40–41.

121. "It is usually agreed": Farmer, "Fresh Ways of Serving Early Fall Fruits," *The Woman's Home Companion*, April 1911, p. 75.

122. In a later article: Farmer, "Dried Fruits," *The Woman's Home Companion*, April 1911, p. 75.

122. "Cupid's Deceits": Demonstration slip, Miss Farmer's School of Cookery, January 31, 1912 (Edith Raymond papers).

122. On St. Patrick's Day: Demonstration slip, Miss Farmer's School of Cookery, February 18, 1914 (Edith Raymond papers).

122. "For a real Christmas": Farmer, "Good Things for the Christmas Dinner," *The Woman's Home Companion*, December 1905, pp. 20–1.

123. "Couldn't it be better": Wilma Lord Perkins to Margo Miller. See also Hartt, "Fannie Merritt Farmer—An Appreciation," p. 21.

123. "Never serve a": Notebook, Lucy Allen papers.

124. six considerations: Farmer, *Food and Cookery for the Sick and Convalescent*, p. 37.

124. "It will suggest": *Ibid.*, p. 182.

124. On December 30, 1914: Demonstration slip, Miss Farmer's School of Cookery, December 30, 1914 (Edith Raymond papers).

125. Her illness was: the *Boston Evening Transcript*, January 15, 1915, p. 1; James, *Notable American Women*, Vol. 1, p. 598.

125. Miss Farmer's estate: Information on Fannie Farmer's estate is from Suffolk County Probate files, provided to me by Margo Miller.

Six

127. a yellow-and-violet dinner: "News from the Field," *New England Kitchen Magazine*, July 1897, pp. 164–5.

127. "Ah!" wrote a: Jones, "Ethics of the Kitchen," p. 110.

128. "It is an interesting fact": Rorer, "Indian Corn Kitchen," *Household News*, October 1893, pp. 121–2.

128. "pickaninnies": *The Woman's Home Companion*, December 1905, pp. 32–3.

128. the "gospel of": See, for example, Jones, "The Ethics of the Kitchen," p. 112 ("Speeding the gospel of good cookery will hasten the triumph of the gospel of redeeming love"). Also, "Cooking Department of the State Farmers Institute," *American Kitchen Magazine*, October 1898, p. 33 ("There are thousands of itinerants in . . . the United States whose whole time is devoted to carrying the gospel of peace to the needy, but only in three or four states have we itinerants going from place to place carrying the gospel of good cooking to the masses . . .").

128. "Schools like these": Letter from Maria Parloa, June 13, 1879, quoted in *Training Schools of Cookery*, p. 32.

128. The sense of mission: See Cott, *The Bonds of Womanhood*; Douglas, *The Feminization of American Culture*; and Keith Melder, *Beginnings of Sisterhood.*

129. "Jane, making a": Mrs. S. S. Robbins, "A Wasted Life," *The Mother at Home and Household Magazine*, May 1869, p. 147.

129. "If we do": Anna C. Pollok, "The Ethical Value of Domestic Science," *American Kitchen Magazine*, April 1899, p. 20.

130. "Compounds like wedding cake": Mary Peabody Mann, *Christianity in the Kitchen*, p. 1.

130. "Chemical analysis": *Ibid.*, p. 10.

131. "foreigners": See Robert A. Woods and Albert J. Kennedy, *Handbook of Settlements*. In this 1911 listing of the country's settlement houses, compiled from information sent by the settlement workers themselves, neighborhood populations are described most commonly as "Americans, Irish, Germans, and Italians" (p. 204) or "Americans, Germans, Hebrews, Italians, Irish, Negroes, Poles, etc." (p. 176).

132. " 'Poor folks can't' ": Campbell, *Darkness and Daylight*, pp. 265–7.

133. "friendly visits": See Mrs. James T. Fields, *How to Help the Poor*; and Mary Richmond, *Friendly Visiting Among the Poor.*

133. "Settlement workers are": Richmond, *Friendly Visiting*, pp. 8, 9.

134. An Irish woman: Campbell, *Darkness and Daylight*, pp. 268–9.

135. "Please send me": Sarah Bolton, *Successful Women*, pp. 24–5.

135. "political demagogues": "The New York Cooking School," *Harper's New Monthly*, December 1879, p. 22.

136. her final illness: *New England Kitchen Magazine*, October 1896, p. 46.

136. "I hope to live": Bolton, *Successful Women*, p. 27.

136. Although she refused: Corson, *Fifteen Cent Dinners for Workingmen's Families*, p. 32.

137. "rough," "gristly": *Ibid.*, p. 10.

137. "savory and nutritious": *Ibid.*, p. v.

137. "What you need": *Ibid.*, p. 20.

137. "sends the man": *Ibid.*, p. v.

137. "The laborer who": Mrs. John A. Logan, "Importance of Domestic and Industrial Training," *Boston Cooking School Magazine*, June–July 1899, p. 10.

137. " 'if we knew' ": Lily A. Toomy, "Wanted—Intelligent Cooks," *New England Kitchen Magazine*, October 1897, p. 11.

138. " 'a cooking school' ": "News from the Field," *New England Kitchen Magazine*, April 1896, p. 50.

138. " 'poor food' ": Atwater, and Charles D. Woods, *Dietary Studies in New York City*, p. 64.

138. "a man is": Quoted in *Training Schools of Cookery*, p. 28. Miss Corson was addressing a convention of Christian women's associations, held in Cleveland in June 1879.

138. "The man who has": Mrs. Helen Ekin Starrett, "The Home and the Labor Problem," *New England Kitchen Magazine*, February 1895, p. 241.

139. "Many of the so-called": Rorer, "Indian Corn Kitchen," *Household News*, October 1893, pp. 121–2.

139. "I am fully persuaded": Mrs. Maude H. Lacy, "A Neglected Side of the Labor Problem," *American Kitchen Magazine*, November 1899, p. 45. Mrs. Lacy read her paper at a meeting of the National Household Economic Association.

139. "It has long": Quoted in Hogan, *History and Present Status of Instruction in Cooking in the Public Schools of New York City*, p. 11.

140. "Our young women": Mary E. Green, "Household Economics," *New England Kitchen Magazine*, January 1897, p. 166.

140. School Kitchen No. 1: Barrows, "The School Kitchens of Boston," *New England Kitchen Magazine*, June–July 1894, p. 138.

141. "a new revelation": *Ibid.*, p. 139.

141. "Skilled cookery": *Idem.*

141. "It is amusing": Angeline M. Weaver, "Incidentals in School Work," *New England Kitchen Magazine*, June–July 1894, p. 145.

142. "the very natural": Barrows, "The School Kitchens of Boston," p. 141.

142. The difference between: *Ibid.*, p. 144.

142. an "antidote": *Ibid.*, p. 145. She was quoting Samuel Capen, a president of the Boston School Board.

143. "One incidental part": Weaver, "Incidentals in School Work," p. 145.

143. "humanized and refined": Barrows, "The School Kitchens of Boston," p. 140. See also Fields, *How to Help the Poor*, p. 49.

143. "dainty daughters": Maria S. Orwig, "A Visit to the Charles Kozminski School of Chicago," *New England Kitchen Magazine*, August 1898, p. 197.

143. "Our little girl": Quoted in Hogan, *History and Present Status of Instruction in Cooking*, p. 35.

144. "without slopping it": Corson, *Cooking School Text Book and Housekeepers' Guide*, p. 54.

144. "tiny crackers": Eliza Noyes Summer, "Recollections of the Atlanta Exposition," *New England Kitchen Magazine*, August 1896, p. 232.

145. "suffer physically": Atwater, "Pecuniary Economy of Food," *The Century*, January 1888, p. 442. See also Atwater, "What We Should Eat," *The Century*, June 1888, p. 260.

145. "To introduce soups": Anna J. Atkinson, "Atlanta University: Student Dietaries," *New England Kitchen Magazine*, July 1896, pp. 162–3.

146. "I went over": Richards, "The Signs of the Times," *New England Kitchen Magazine*, December 1895, p. 104.

146. "Thus we ensured": Mrs. E. C. Hobson, "Industrial Education for Women in the South," a paper presented at the Chautauqua, New York, Assembly, July–August 1896. Reported in "The Domestic Economy Conference," *New England Kitchen Magazine*, November 1896, p. 73.

147. the "refinements of": Alice C. Hewett, "The Work of the 'Field Matron' Among Indian Women," *New England Kitchen Magazine*, March 1898, p. 216.

147. "crisp, brown loaves": "Home Science Among the North Dakota Indian," *New England Kitchen Magazine*, February 1897, p. 221.

147. "The primitive manner": *Teaching the Rudiments of Cooking in the Class Room*, pp. 45, 32.

149. the "food and nutrition": Hunt, *The Life of Ellen H. Richards*, p. 215.

149. "a mess of": Edward Atkinson, *The Science of Nutrition*, p. 13.

150. "At the extraordinary": *Ibid.*, p. 40.

150. "persons of very moderate intelligence": Atkinson, "The Right Application of Heat to the Conversion of Food Material," *Proceedings of the American Association for the Advancement of Science, for the 39th Meeting*, pp. 413–30.

150. "I do not fancy": Atkinson, *The Science of Nutrition*, p. 35.

151. "distasteful to women": Letter, Ellen Richards to Edward Atkinson, February 12, 1892.

151. "We believe this": Reported in Atkinson, "The Right Application of Heat," pp. 417, 419.

152. "Good Food for Little Money": Mary Hinman Abel, in *Plain Words About Food*, p. 129.

153. "Even a casual": Isabel Bevier, *Home Economics in Education*, pp. 191–2.

153. "All observing travelers": Abel, *Practical Sanitary and Economic Cooking Adapted to Persons of Moderate and Small Means*, p. 15.

153. "flour pancakes": *Ibid.*, p. 151.

153. "I only ask": *Ibid.*, p. 146.

154. Beef broth: Richards, "Scientific Cooking-Studies in the New England Kitchen," *The Forum*, May 1893, pp. 356–7; and Maria Parloa, "The New England Kitchen," *The Century*, December 1891, p. 316.

154. "Certainly we are": Letters, Ellen Richards to Edward Atkinson, March 8, 1890, and June 25, 1890.

155. "Between eleven and": Parloa, "The New England Kitchen," pp. 315–17.

156. "a fitting place": "The Rumford Kitchen at the World's Fair," *New England Kitchen Magazine*, April 1894, p. 11.

156. "Wherefore do you": "Rumford Kitchen Mottoes," in *Plain Words About Food*, pp. 16–18.

156. "I propose to": Letter, Ellen Richards to Edward Atkinson, May 11, 1893. See also "The Rumford Kitchen at the World's Fair," p. 11.

156. "owing to certain": Richards, "Count Rumford, and His Work for Humanity," *New England Kitchen Magazine*, March 1898, p. 203. For a more detached view of Count Rumford's life, see Duane Bradley, *Count Rumford*, and Egon Larson, *An American in Europe*.

156. "the King of England": Richards, "Count Rumford," p. 204.

158. "It was without": Bradley, p. 165.

158. Mrs. Richards calculated: Richards, "Count Rumford," p. 205.

158. "puzzle and repel": "Count Rumford and the New England Kitchen," *New England Kitchen Magazine*, April 1894, p. 7.

158. "It was disheartening": Richards, "Scientific Cooking-Studies," p. 357.

159. "Those who come": Abel, "The Story of the New England Kitchen," in *Plain Words About Food*, pp. 139–50.

160. "The person who said": *Ibid.*, p. 159.

160. "The taste of the": Letter, Edward Atkinson to T. A. Havemeyer, February 19, 1894.

161. "No better school": Richards, "Hospital Diet," *New England Kitchen Magazine*, April 1894, p. 22.

161. an "atmosphere of": *Idem.*

162. "Perhaps the treatment": Carroll D. Wright, *The Italians in Chicago*, p. 46.

162. "The increased interest": "Dietaries for Public Institutions," *New England Kitchen Magazine*, August 1897, p. 188.

162. Prisoners, she instructed: *Ibid.*, p. 189.

163. "personal idiosyncrasies": *Ibid.*, p. 191.

164. the "pecuniary economy": Atwater, "The Pecuniary Economy of Food," *The Century*, January 1888, p. 437.

164. "Eternal vigilance": Bevier, "The U.S. Government and the Housewife," *American Kitchen Magazine*, December 1898, p. 78.

165. the "solid excreta": Atwater, Bulletin 21, p. 203.

165. a "frank talk": Bevier, "The U.S. Government and the Housewife," p. 79.

165. In one Pittsburgh family: Bevier, "Nutrition Investigations in Pittsburgh, Pa., 1894–1896," U.S. Department of Agriculture, Bulletin 52, pp. 22–7.

166. "per man per day": See Atwater, Bulletin 21, p. 199; and Atwater and Woods, *Dietary Studies in New York City in 1895 and 1896*, U.S. Department of Agriculture, Bulletin 46, pp. 5–7, for Atwater's description of his methods.

167. The only designations: Atwater, Bulletin 21, p. 213.

167. black tenant farmers: Atwater and Woods, *Dietary Studies with Reference to the Food of the Negro in Alabama in 1895 and 1896*, U.S. Department of Agriculture, Bulletin 38, p. 23.

167. done in New York City: Atwater and Woods, *Dietary Studies in New York City*, pp. 12, 45–7, 49.

168. "from Maine to Oregon": Campbell, "Household Science as a University Movement," *New England Kitchen Magazine*, November 1894, pp. 54–5.

168. "bruised and weary pilgrims": *Ibid.*, p. 58.

Seven

169. some of her dreams: Richards, "Housekeeping in the Twentieth Century," *American Kitchen Magazine*, March 1900, pp. 203–7.

171. "steak & chops": Letter, Ellen Richards to Edward Atkinson, November 15, 1899.

171. the "leaven of progress": Richards, *The Cost of Shelter*, p. 8.

171. the "majority": Richards, *The Cost of Living*, p. 3.

171. the "class to work": Richards, *The Cost of Shelter*, p. 8.

171. "sane and wholesome living": *Ibid.*, p. 9.

171. "Tom and Sally": Rose Terry Cooke, "Tom and Sally," *Good Housekeeping*, May 30, 1885, pp. 6–7.

173. "Chocolate cake": Campbell, "Household Science as a University Movement," p. 54.

173. Much to Edward Atkinson's: Atkinson, "Home Life: Why Not?" *New England Kitchen Magazine*, January 1897, pp. 145–7. ("I have devoted my leisure time for ten or twelve years, spent a lot of money and after going all round a simple problem in a most complex and devious way, I have at length placed an oven . . . at the disposal of woman . . . The comforts of good cooking . . . are all assured at the least cost. Why cannot men enjoy them? Because *women* won't have them.")

174. "It is usually": Barrows, "Foes in Our Own Household," *New England Kitchen Magazine*, January 1898, pp. 123–6. Miss Barrows read her paper at the annual meeting of the NHEA in Nashville.

174. "incoherent primitiveness": Campbell, *Household Economics*, pp. xi–ii.

175. "Women have lacked": Quoted in Barrows, "Foes in Our Own Household," p. 124.

175. an apologetic letter: Letter, Kate M. Cone to Ellen Richards, February 24, 1902.

175. "Make us seriously enthusiastic": Letter, Caroline Hunt to Ellen Richards, October 28, 1907.

175. "Please do not": Letter, M. Carey Thomas to Ellen Richards, November 1, 1907.

176. "could never expect": Proceedings of the first Lake Placid Conference, p. 5.

177. The word "home": Quoted in Hunt, *The Life of Ellen H. Richards*, p. 268.

178. a "lack of attention": "Home Economics, the Lake Placid Conference," *American Kitchen Magazine*, November 1899, p. 68.

178. "Let us remember": Henrietta Goodrich, "Suggestion for a Professional School of Home and Social Economics," *American Kitchen Magazine*, September 1900, p. 208.

179. she was "astounded": M. Carey Thomas, "Present Tendencies in Women's College and University Education," *Publications of the Association of Collegiate Alumnae*, February 1908, pp. 45–62.

180. "those lines of thought": Mary Roberts Smith, "Shall the College Curriculum be Modified for Women?" *Publications of the Association of Collegiate Alumnae*, December 1898, pp. 1–15.

180. a systematic course of study: Goodrich, "Suggestion for a Professional School," pp. 199–208.

181. "That is why": Richards, *The Cost of Living*, pp. 137–8.

181. "The cost of living": Proceedings of the first Lake Placid conference, p. 6.

181. the "germ of": Richards, *The Cost of Living*, p. 5.

181. "I thought I had": Quoted in Lita Bane, *The Story of Isabel Bevier*, p. 29.

182. the "place for": *Ibid.*, p. 45.
182. "and thus due": *Ibid.*, p. 35.
182. "The courses were": *Ibid.*, p. 39.
183. "the first woman": *Ibid.*, p. 52.
184. "and to my joy": *Ibid.*, pp. 50–1.
184. "the age-old conflict": *Ibid.*, p. 53.
185. "well-intentioned": *Ibid.*, p. 58.
185. "It is here": *Ibid.*, p. 59.
185. "it seems as if": Bevier, *Home Economics in Education*, p. 93.

186. "other courses": Charles Van Hise, "Educational Tendencies in State Universities," *Publications of the Association of Collegiate Alumnae*, February 1908, pp. 31–43.

187. "When the boys": Nellie S. Kedzie, "The Teaching of Domestic Science in an Agricultural College," *University Magazine*, n.d., pp. 94–8 (probably ca. 1894).

187. In some universities: A. C. True, *A History of Agricultural Education in the United States, 1785–1925*, p. 271.

188. "cooking tiny bits": Bane, pp. 168–9.

188. "household joy": Charles W. Eliot, "Woman's Education—A Forecast," *Publications of the Association of Collegiate Alumnae*, February 1908, p. 101–5.

188. "Neither pious intentions": Bevier, *Home Economics in Education*, p. 188.

189. "peace and restfulness": Richards, "Housekeeping in the Twentieth Century," p. 204.

189. "But of one thing": Anna C. Pollak, "The Ethical Value of Domestic Science," *New England Kitchen Magazine*, April 1899, p. 21.

189. blunt little story: Campbell, "A Club Episode," *Boston Cooking School Magazine*, February 1904, pp. 340–2.

190. "It was one": Campbell, "Household Science as a University Movement," p. 55.

Eight

191. "We made a": *The Woman's Home Companion*, February 1911, p. 50 (Quaker Oats); *The Woman's Home Companion*, December 1904, p. 50 (Domino Sugar); *Boston Cooking School Magazine*, March 1902, p. xi (Heinz Baked Beans); *The Woman's Home Companion*, March 1910, p. 63 (Baker's Cocoa); *The Woman's Home Companion*, June 1910, p. 43 (Van Camp's Pork and Beans); *The Woman's Home Companion*, July 1910, p. 22 (Campbell's Tomato Soup).

192. their modern form: See Richard Cummings, *The American and His Food*; and Susan Strasser, *Never Done*.

192. active commercial careers: See Emma Weigley, *Sarah Tyson Rorer*, pp. 38–41.

193. "After a *careful*": Quoted in Weigley, p. 42.

194. "A Bright Galaxy": *New England Kitchen Magazine*, May 1894, inside back cover.

194. desiccated codfish: Harland, *Common Sense in the Household*, p. 52.

194. Red Robin Pudding: The recipe first appeared in "Recipes from Public Demonstrations—Boston Cooking School," *Boston Cooking School Magazine*, June–July 1902, p. 34. The query and explanation appeared in "Queries and Answers," *Boston Cooking School Magazine*, October 1902, p. 141.

195. "There are many ways": Lincoln, editorial, *American Kitchen Magazine*, July 1899, pp. 157–8.

196. "absolutely injurious": "Grocery News," *Table Talk*, February 1888, p. 92.

196. "housekeeper's laboratory": Richards, "The Housekeeper's Laboratory," *New England Kitchen Magazine*, April 1895, pp. 5–6.

196. the "average housekeeper": Mary Caldwell, "Food Adulterations," *American Kitchen Magazine*, November 1898, pp. 60–63.

197. "The practices which": "Food Fairs," *New England Kitchen Magazine*, October 1894, p. 43.

197. an enterprising sideline: See, for example, Rorer, "The Cleveland Food Exposition," *Household News*, May 1894, p. 463. ("We move on from city to city, leaving each place, as Ruskin tells us we should, as though we had intended to remain our life-time . . . And now we move on to Detroit, where, we are told, the cream of charming people resides.") See also "Grand Rapids, Mich., Food Exposition," *Household News*, July 1894, p. 580. ("As we leave Grand Rapids we feel that we are leaving behind many new but true friends. We ride west to Butte, where again new faces will appear to disappear, as those before.")

198. "One could not": "Chicago's Pure Food Exposition," *New England Kitchen Magazine*, November 1894, p. 64.

198. exposition of 1892: Mrs. M. C. Myer, "Philadelphia Food Exposition," *Table Talk*, January 1893, pp. 33–7.

199. a Boston exposition: "World's Food Fair," *New England Kitchen Magazine*, October 1894, pp. 3–10.

199. "Surely a philanthropic work": Myer, "Philadelphia Food Exposition," p. 33.

199. the "business adventurer": "World's Food Fair," p. 3.

200. "dainty and beautiful": "The Home Department: Boston Food Fair," *New England Kitchen Magazine*, October 1894, p. 59.

200. decorative table settings: "World's Food Fair," p. 9.

200. a Hygienic Lunch: : "The Home Department," pp. 61–3.

201. "the influence of": "World's Food Fair," p. 3.

201. "Once more we": Rorer, "The Cleveland Food Exposition," p. 463.

201. "Those who can": Lincoln, "From Cottage and Cave," *American Kitchen Magazine*, March 1902, p. 211.

202. "A dainty dish": *Boston Cooking School Magazine*, March 1902, p. xi.

202. no literary person: Rorer, "Mrs. Rorer's Answers to Questions," *Ladies' Home Journal*, February 1897, p. 32.

202. Bean Celery Salad: *The Woman's Home Companion*, November 1912, p. 53. A baked bean salad made with home-baked beans had been offered a decade earlier (Morrill, "Winter Salads," *American Kitchen Magazine*, March 1903, p. 232) but to little avail.

202. "No person would": Barrows, "Emergency Dinners," *New England Kitchen Magazine*, June 1898, p. 101.

203. "hands do not": Christine Terhune Herrick, "What I Have Learned About Canned Foods," *The Woman's Home Companion*, February 1914, p. 20.

204. "Why, we never": *The Woman's Home Companion*, November 1912, p. 53.

204. "beefsteak tomato ketchup": See Cornelia C. Bedford, "New Menus for August," *Table Talk*, August 1899, pp. 300–1; and Bedford, "New Menus for October," *Table Talk*, October 1902, pp. 279–80.

204. catsup with sherry: Rorer, "Our Bills of Fare," *Household News*, November 1894, p. 715.

204. fricasseed partridges: Lincoln, "From Day to Day," *New England Kitchen Magazine*, October 1895, p. 32.

204. French dressing: Farmer, "Good Salads for Summer," *The Woman's Home Companion*, July 1911, p. 35.

204. "When opened the banana": Marian C. Keller, "Cold Dishes for Hot Days," *Boston Cooking School Magazine*, June–July 1913, p. 50.

204. baked cream-cheese: Farmer, *A New Book of Cookery*, p. 389.

204. grapefruit halves: *Ibid.*, p. 392.

205. pieces of marshmallow: Ibid., pp. 208–9.

205. Ginger Ale Salad: Farmer, "A February Luncheon Menu," *The Woman's Home Companion*, February 1912, p. 48.

205. Even gingerbread: Farmer, "A Dozen Good Desserts," *The Woman's Home Companion*, May 1912, p. 60.

205. old-fashioned treat: Virginia Church, "Sue Breckinridge Invites the Veranda Girls to a Mid-Winter Picnic," *Boston Cooking School Magazine*, January 1912, p. 297.

205. "I usually go": Ellen Marshall Rugg, in Susie Root Rhodes and Grace Porter Hopkins, *The Economy Administration Cook Book*, p. 246.

206. plain cake (No. 1): Reprinted in Alice Ravenhill, *The Teaching of "Domestic Science" in the United States of America*, pp. 157–8.

208. chart for cupcakes: "Book Reviews," *New England Kitchen Magazine*, August 1894, p. 254.

209. "Typical Correctly": Emma Jacobs, "How to Plan Meals," *The Journal of Home Economics*, April 1911, pp. 162–7.

210. "home cooking as": Massachusetts Bureau of Statistics and Labor, *Comparison of the Cost of Home-Made and Prepared Food*, p. 31.

211. fancy cookie cutters: Barrows and Lincoln, *The Home Science Cook Book*, p. 207.

211. frosting sandwich: "Household Hints," *Boston Cooking School Magazine*, April–May 1898, n.p.

211. glacé cherries: "Public Demonstrations from Boston Cooking School," *Boston Cooking School Magazine*, March 1902, p. 373.

211–12. bananas and pimentos: Hill, *Practical Cooking and Serving*, pp. 352, 364.

212. dinner so orderly: "White House Menus," Rhodes and Hopkins, *The Economy Administration Cook Book*, p. 42.

212. "Americans do not": George E. Walsh, "Queer Foreign Foods in America," *America Kitchen Magazine*, October 1901, p. 65.

212. Indian and Sinhalese: Weigley, *Sarah Tyson Rorer*, p. 96.

212. "Hindoo": Campbell, "Some East Indian Ways with American Vegetables," *Boston Cooking School Magazine*, February–March 1900, pp. 207–10.

212. Chinese Eggs: Rorer, "Answers to Inquiries," *Household News*, August 1894, p. 589.

212. "Japanese luncheon": "Menu for Japanese Luncheon," in "Queries and Answers," *Boston Cooking-School Magazine*, March 1904, p. 426.

213. "intellectual merits": Hartford Beaumont, "A Japanese Restaurant," *American Kitchen Magazine*, July 1902, pp. 146–7.

213. "local tastes and": "Standards of Living as Interpreted Thru Facts in Regard to Food," Proceedings of the fourth Lake Placid conference, pp. 39–44.

214. "the great bakeries": Caroline Hunt, "Tendencies Toward Public and Private Industries in Woman's Work," Proceedings of the fourth Lake Placid conference, pp. 44–7.

214. "An Absolutely New Product": *The Woman's Home Companion*, January 1912, p. 39.

215. Caramel Sweet Potatoes: *Vegetable Cookery*, pp. 10, 12, 15; and *School Lunches*, p. 18.

216. "The final goal": Bane, *The Story of Isabel Bevier*, p. 184.

Conclusion

218. "It nearly killed": Bevier, "Reconstruction Days in Home Economics," *The Journal of Home Economics*, August 1922, p. 362.

219. effectively barred: See, for example, the entries for Kath-

arine Blunt, Hazel Kyrk, and Agnes Fay Morgan in Sicherman and Green, *Notable American Women.*

220. "there is evidence": Chase Going Woodhouse, *Business Opportunities for the Home Economist*, pp. 15–16.

221. "Our basic products": Marjorie Hostetter, "How I Use My Experimental Kitchen," Parts I and II, *American Kitchen Magazine*, December 1946, pp. 41–2, 56; and January 1947, pp. 16–17, 60.

222. day-to-day work: See Strasser, *Never Done.*

223. "curiously happy and provocative": Margaret Culkin Banning, "Love Flies Out of the Kitchen," *Ladies' Home Journal*, January 1933, pp. 3–4, 50–1.

224. "The results of": Mariana T. Nelson, "What Homemakers Learned About Purchasing Household Goods," *The Journal of Home Economics*, June 1932, pp. 519–20.

224. "Such advertising": Ruth Atwater, "Information About Canned Food Products," *The Journal of Home Economics*, June 1932, pp. 527–9.

225. " 'I don't like housework!' ": *Ladies' Home Journal*, February 1938, p. 57.

225. "Lack of the": Elizabeth Macdonald and Forrester Macdonald, *Homemaking, A Profession for Men and Women*, p. 204.

225. "is thrown into": Emily Newell Blair, *The Creation of a Home*, p. 187.

226. "something of its": Susan F. West, "The Education of Women for Leisure," *The Journal of Home Economics*, p. 495.

226. "Amy was largely": Paul Popenoe, "Can This Marriage Be Saved?" *Ladies' Home Journal*, May 1953, p. 60.

226. " 'I hear' ": Louise Paine Benjamin, "Under Thirty," *Ladies' Home Journal*, June 1938, p. 35.

227. " 'My difficult darling' ": Dale Carnegie, "Who's Boss in Your Home?" *Woman's Day*, November 1937, p. 5.

227. "You all know": William G. Niederland, "Some Psychological Disorders of Femininity and Masculinity," *Women, Society, and Sex*, p. 98.

227. " 'I'll be there!' ": *Ladies' Home Journal*, August 1942, p. 35.

228. "Learn to cook": "Tryouts for the Young Bride," *Ladies' Home Journal*, May 1953, p. 164.

229. "Cut 2 boxes": "31 Money-Saving Menus for March," *Woman's Day*, March 1958, p. 70.

233. Back in 1903: Marion Harland, *Marion Harland's Complete Cook Book*, p. 144.

234. ". . . a glass dish": Pryse, ed., "A New England Nun," in *Selected Stories of Mary E. Wilkins Freeman*, pp. 109–25.

236. "a source of": Woman's Education Association Annual Report, 1884, p. 12.

Bibliography

Abel, Mary Hinman. "Practical Experiments for the Promotion of Home Economics." *The Journal of Home Economics*, October 1911, pp. 362–9.

———. *Practical Sanitary and Economic Cooking Adapted to Persons of Moderate and Small Means* (Rochester: The American Public Health Association, 1890).

Addams, Jane. "The Subtle Problems of Charity." *The Atlantic*, February 1899, pp. 163–78.

———. *Twenty Years at Hull-House* (New York: Phillips Publishing Co., 1910).

Alcott, Louisa May. *An Old-Fashioned Girl* (Boston: Little, Brown, 1870).

———. *Work* (New York: Schocken Books, 1977).

Andrews, Benjamin R. *Current Progress in Education for the Home* (Washington, D.C.: Government Printing Office, 1915).

Aresty, Esther B. *The Delectable Past* (New York: Bobbs-Merrill, 1964).

Armstrong, Florence. "Managerial Status of Women in Food Service and Institutional Housekeeping." *The Journal of Home Economics*, April 1932, pp. 340–2.

Atkinson, Edward. "The Right Application of Heat to the Conversion of Food Material." *Proceedings of the American Association for the Advancement of Science*, August 1890, pp. 413–30.

———. *The Science of Nutrition* (Boston: Damrell and Upham, 1896).

———. *Suggestions for the Establishment of Food Laboratories in Connection with the Agricultural Experiment Stations of the United States* (Washington, D.C.: Government Printing Office, 1893).

Atwater, Ruth. "Information about Canned Food Products." *The Journal of Home Economics*, June 1932, pp. 527–9.

Atwater, W. O. "The Composition of Our Bodies and Our Food." *The Century*, May 1887, pp. 59–74.

———. "The Digestibility of Food." *The Century*, September 1887, pp. 733–40.

———. "The Food Supply of the Future." *The Century*, November 1891, pp. 101–12.

———. *Foods: Nutritive Value and Cost* (Washington, D.C.: Government Printing Office, 1894).

———. "How Food Nourishes the Body." *The Century*, June 1887, pp. 237–51.

———. *Methods and Results of Investigations of the Chemistry and*

Economy of Food (Washington, D.C.: Government Printing Office, 1895).

———. "Pecuniary Economy of Food." *The Century*, January 1888, pp. 437–46.

———. "The Potential Energy of Food." *The Century*, July 1887, pp. 397–405.

———. "What We Should Eat." *The Century*, June 1888, pp. 257–64.

Atwater, W. O., and A. P. Bryant. *Dietary Studies in Chicago in 1895 and 1896* (Washington, D.C.: Government Printing Office, 1898).

Atwater, W. O., and Charles Woods. *The Chemical Composition of American Food Materials* (Washington, D.C.: Government Printing Office, 1896).

———. *Dietary Studies in New York City in 1895 and 1896* (Washington, D.C.: Government Printing Office, 1898).

———. *Dietary Studies with Reference to the Food of the Negro in Alabama in 1895 and 1896* (Washington, D.C.: Government Printing Office, 1897).

Baldwin, Keturah. *The AHEA Saga* (Washington, D.C.: The American Home Economics Association, 1949).

Bane, Lita. "Major Objectives in Home Economics." *The Journal of Home Economics*, March 1927, pp. 119–22.

———. *The Story of Isabel Bevier* (Peoria: Chas. A. Bennett Co., 1955).

Banner, Lois W. *Women in Modern America* (New York: Harcourt Brace Jovanovich, 1974).

Barber, Solon. "Tricky Labels on Foods." *The Journal of Home Economics*, June 1932, pp. 502–6.

Barrows, Anna. *Principles of Cookery* (Chicago: American School of Home Economics, 1907).

Barrows, Anna, and Mary J. Lincoln. *The Home Science Cook Book* (Boston: Whitcomb and Barrows, 1902).

Barrows, Anna, and Bertha E. Shapleigh. *An Outline on the History of Cookery* (New York: Teachers College, Columbia University, 1917).

Baym, Nina. *Woman's Fiction* (Ithaca: Cornell University Press, 1978).

Beecher, Catharine. "How to Redeem Woman's Profession from Dishonor." *Harper's New Monthly Magazine*, November 1865, pp. 710–16.

———. *Miss Beecher's Domestic Receipt Book* (New York: Harper and Brothers, 1846).

———. *Miss Beecher's Housekeeper and Healthkeeper* (New York: Harper and Brothers, 1874).

———. *A Treatise on Domestic Economy* (New York: Marsh Capen Lyon and Webb, 1841).

———. "Woman's Profession Dishonored." *Harper's New Monthly Magazine*, November 1864, pp. 766–8.

Beecher, Catharine, and Harriet Beecher Stowe. *The American Woman's Home* (New York: J. B. Ford and Co., 1869).

———. *Principles of Domestic Science* (New York: J. B. Ford and Co., 1873).

Betters, Paul V. *The Bureau of Home Economics* (Washington, D.C.: The Brookings Institution, 1930).

Bevier, Isabel. *Home Economics in Education* (Philadelphia: J. B. Lippincott, 1924).

———. *Nutrition Investigations in Pittsburgh, Pa., 1894–1896* (Washington, D.C.: Government Printing Office, 1898).

———. *The Planning of Meals* (Urbana: Department of Household Science, University of Illinois, 1914).

———. "Reconstruction Days in Home Economics." *The Journal of Home Economics*, August 1922, pp. 361–3.

———. *Some Points in the Making and Judging of Bread* (Urbana: Department of Household Science, University of Illinois, 1913).

Bevier, Isabel, and Susannah Usher. *The Home Economics Movement* (Boston: Whitcomb and Barrows, 1906).

Blair, Emily Newell. *The Creation of a Home* (New York: Farrar and Rinehart, 1930).

Blair, Karen J. *The Clubwoman as Feminist* (New York: Holmes and Meier, 1980).

Blot, Pierre. *Hand-Book of Practical Cookery* (New York: Appleton and Co., 1884).

———. *Lectures on Cookery* (Boston, 186–).

Bok, Edward. *The Americanization of Edward Bok* (New York: Scribner's, 1922).

Bolton, Sarah K. *Successful Women* (Boston: D. Lothrop, 1888).

"The Boston Cooking School." Leaflet, 1882.

Boston Cooking School Committee. Minutes of the Meetings (manuscript notebook, Simmons College Archives).

Bradley, Duane. *Count Rumford* (New York: D. Van Nostrand, 1967).

Brown, Sanborn C., ed. *The Collected Works of Count Rumford* (Cambridge, Mass.: Harvard University Press, 1968).

Brumbert, Joan Jacobs. "Chlorotic Girls, 1870–1920: A Historical Perspective on Female Adolescence." *Child Development*, 1982, 53, pp. 1468–77.

"Business and Information for the Consumer." *The Journal of Home Economics*, January 1932, pp. 40–2.

Byington, Margaret. *Homestead* (Pittsburgh: University of Pittsburgh, 1974).

Calvin, Henrietta W., and Carrie A. Lyford. *Home Economics, 1916* (Washington, D.C.: Government Printing Office, 1916).

Campbell, Helen. *Darkness and Daylight; or Lights and Shadows of New York Life* (Hartford: A. D. Worthington, 1892).

———. *Household Economics* (New York: G. P. Putnam's Sons, 1896).

Child, Lydia Maria. *The American Frugal Housewife* (Boston: Carter Hendee and Co., 1833).

Clark, Ava Milam, and J. Kenneth Munford. *Adventures of a Home Economist* (Corvallis: Oregon State University Press, 1969).

Clarke, Robert. *Ellen Swallow* (Chicago: Follett, 1973).

Combe, Andrew. *The Physiology of Digestion* (New York: William H. Colyer, 1846).

Cone, Kate M. *Publications of the Association of Collegiate Alumnae*, 1898, pp. 32–5.

Congdon, Leon A. *Fight for Food* (Philadelphia: J. B. Lippincott, 1916).

Conway, Jill. "Women Reformers and American Culture 1870–1930." *Journal of Social History*, Winter 1971–2, pp. 164–77.

Corson, Juliet. *Cooking School Text Book; and Housekeepers' Guide to Cookery and Kitchen Management* (New York: Orange Judd Co., 1879).

———. *A Course of Lectures on the Principles of Domestic Economy and Cookery* (St. Paul: The Pioneer Press Co., 1887).

———. *Fifteen Cent Dinners for Workingmen's Families* (New York: 1877).

Cott, Nancy F. *The Bonds of Womanhood* (New Haven: Yale University Press, 1977).

"Course of Instruction at the Boston Cooking School." Pamphlet, n.d., probably 1884.

Cummings, Richard Osborn. *The American and His Food* (Chicago: University of Chicago Press, 1940).

Curtis, Lucy. "Fannie Farmer's Life Story One of Magnificent Courage." *The Boston Herald*, September 8, 1947.

Dainty Desserts for Dainty People (Johnstown, N.Y.: Charles B. Knox Gelatine Company, Inc., 1927).

Dame, L. M. "The Relation of Diet to School-Life." A paper presented to the Association of Collegiate Alumnae on October 30, 1886.

Davis, Allen F. *American Heroine* (New York: Oxford University Press, 1978).

Degler, Carl. *At Odds* (New York: Oxford University Press, 1980).

Desserts (Cincinnati: Procter & Gamble Co., 1926).

Dewey, Mary E., ed. *Life & Letters of Catharine M. Sedgwick* (New York: Harper & Bros., 1871).

Dewey, Melvil. *Decimal Classification and Relativ Index* (Lake Placid Club, N.Y.: Forest Press, 1911).

Donham, S. Agnes. *The Eastern Massachusetts Home Economics Association, Formerly the New England Home Economics*

Association, The First Forty-Three Years, 1909–1952 (Eastern Massachusetts Home Economics Association, 1954).

Douglas, Ann. *The Feminization of American Culture* (New York: Knopf, 1977).

Driscoll, Betty. "Farmer School of Cookery Locates Kitchen of Its Own." *The Christian Science Monitor*, April 30, 1949.

DuBois, Ellen Carol. *Feminism and Suffrage* (Ithaca: Cornell University Press, 1978).

Eagle, Mary Kavanaugh Oldham, ed. *The Congress of Women* (Chicago: American Publishing House, 1894).

Eaves, Lucile. *The Food of Working Women in Boston* (Boston: Wright and Potter Printing Co., 1917).

Ehrenreich, Barbara, and Deirdre English. *For Her Own Good* (New York: Doubleday, 1978).

Everett, Ruth. "Teaching the Homemakers." *Munsey's Magazine*, January 1904, pp. 491–3.

Ewen, Stuart. *Captains of Consciousness* (New York: McGraw-Hill, 1976).

Fairchild, J. E., ed. *Women, Society & Sex* (New York: Fawcett, 1956).

Faithfull, Emily. *Three Visits to America* (Edinburgh: David Douglas, 1884).

Farmer, Fannie. *A Book of Good Dinners for My Friend*, or *What to Have for Dinner* (New York: Dodge, 1905).

———. *The Boston Cooking-School Cook Book* (Boston: Little, Brown, 1896). (Revised editions, 1906, 1918, 1923, 1930, 1941, 1965.)

———. *Catering for Special Occasions* (Philadelphia: David McKay, 1911).

———. *Food and Cookery for the Sick and Convalescent* (Boston: Little, Brown, 1907).

———. *A New Book of Cookery* (Boston: Little, Brown, 1912).

Fields, Mrs. James T. *How to Help the Poor* (Boston: Houghton Mifflin, 1884).

Filippini, Alessandro. *The Table* (New York: Charles L. Webster, 1890).

First Annual Report of the Boston Cooking School (Boston: Mills, Knight, 1884).

Fischer, Christiane, ed. *Let Them Speak for Themselves.* (Hamden, Conn.: Archon Books, 1977).

Flexner, Eleanor. *Century of Struggle* (Cambridge, Mass.: Harvard University Press, 1975).

Francke, Marie. *Opportunities for Women in Domestic Science* ([Philadelphia] Association of Collegiate Alumnae, 1916).

Frankfort, Roberta. *Collegiate Women* (New York: New York University Press, 1977).

Frederick, Christine. Papers (manuscript, Schlesinger Library, Radcliffe College).

Funk, Casimir, and H. E. Dubin. *History of the Discovery of Vitamins* (New York: U.S. Vitamin Corp., 1936).

Gawler, Mrs. Joseph C. "The Home Within and Without." *Journal of Home Economics*, November 1922, pp. 568–9.

Giedion, Siegfried. *Mechanization Takes Command* (New York: Oxford University Press, 1948).

Gilbreth, Frank B. *Primer of Scientific Management* (New York: D. Van Nostrand, 1912).

Gilman, Stella Scott. *Mothers in Council* (New York: Harper and Bros., 1884).

Goodenough, Lizzie A. Wilson. Diary, 1865–1874(?) (manuscript, American Antiquarian Association).

Gordon, Linda. *Woman's Body, Woman's Right* (New York: Grossman/Viking, 1976).

Greenough, Marietta. Papers (manuscript, Houghton Library, Harvard University).

Harland, Marion. *Common Sense in the Household* (New York: Scribner's, 1871).

———. *The Dinner Year-Book* (New York: Scribner's, 1878).

———. *Marion Harland's Complete Cook Book* (St. Louis: The Marion Company, 1903).

Hartman, Mary S., and Lois Banner. *Clio's Consciousness Raised* (New York: Harper and Row, 1974).

Hartt, Mary Bronson. "Fannie Merritt Farmer—An Appreciation." *The Woman's Home Companion*, December 1915, p. 21.

Hayden, Dolores. *The Grand Domestic Revolution* (Cambridge Mass.: MIT Press, 1981).

———. *Redesigning the American Dream* (New York: Norton, 1984).

Hembre, Mrs. Cora Lanning. "The Mother's Part in Teaching Home Economics." *Journal of Home Economics*, June 1927, pp. 316–9.

Herrick, Christine Terhune. *The New Idea Home and Cook Book* (New York: Isaac H. Blanchard and Co., 1900).

Hess, John L., and Karen Hess. *The Taste of America* (New York: Viking/Grossman, 1977).

Hill, Janet McKenzie. *Practical Cooking and Serving* (New York: Doubleday, Page and Co., 1902).

———. *The Whys of Cooking* (Cincinnati: The Procter & Gamble Co., 1916).

Hills, J. L., and Charles E. Wait and H. C. White. *Dietary Studies in Rural Regions in Vermont, Tennessee and Georgia* (Washington, D.C.: Government Printing Office, 1909).

Hogan, Louise E. *History and Present Status of Instruction in Cooking in the Public Schools of New York City* (Washington, D.C.: Government Printing Office, 1899).

"The Home Economics Movement in the United States." *The Journal of Home Economics*, October 1911, pp. 323–41.

Hunt, Caroline. *Home Problems from a New Standpoint* (Boston: Whitcomb and Barrows, 1908).

———. *The Life of Ellen H. Richards* (Boston: Whitcomb and Barrows, 1918).

Huret, Jules. *En Amérique* (Paris: Bibliothèque Charpentier, 1904).

Inter-Municipal Committee on Household Research. Bulletins, November 1904–May 1906.

Jackson, Edith Talbot. "Thrift in the Kitchen from the European Standpoint." *The Journal of Home Economics*, April 1911, pp. 126–30.

Jacobs, Emma S. "How to Plan Meals." *The Journal of Home Economics*, April 1911, pp. 162–7.

Jaffa, Adele S. *A Standard Dietary for an Orphanage* (Sacramento: California State Printing Office, 1915).

James, Edward T., ed. *Notable American Women*, volumes I, II, III (Cambridge, Mass.: Harvard University Press, 1971).

Jesse, R. H. "The Position of Household Economics in the Academic Curriculum." Publications of the Association of Collegiate Alumnae, January, 1905, pp. 24–9.

Johnson, Allen, ed. *Dictionary of American Biography* (New York: Scribner's, 1928).

Jones, Evan. *American Food* (New York: Dutton, 1975).

Katzman, David M. *Seven Days a Week* (Urbana: University of Illinois Press, 1978).

Kedzie, Nellie. "The Teaching of Domestic Science in an Agricultural College." *University Magazine*, n.d. (probably 1894), pp. 94–8.

Keech, Mabel Louise. *Training the Little Home Maker* (Philadelphia: J. B. Lippincott Co., 1912).

Kelley, Mary. "The Sentimentalists: Promise and Betrayal in the Home." *Signs*, Spring 1979, pp. 434–46.

———. ed. *Woman's Being, Woman's Place* (Boston: G. K. Hall, 1979).

Kraditor, Aileen S., ed. *Up from the Pedestal* (New York: Quadrangle, 1968).

Langworthy, C. F. "Food and Diet in the United States." *Yearbook of the United States Department of Agriculture*, pp. 361–78 (Washington, D.C.: Government Printing Office, 1908).

———. *Food Customs and Diet in American Homes* (Washington, D.C.: Government Printing Office, 1911).

———. "Origin and Development of the Nutrition Investigations of the Office of Experiment Stations." *Annual Reports of the Office of Experiment Stations*, pp. 449–60 (Washington, D.C.: Government Printing Office, 1911).

Larsen, Egon. *An American in Europe* (London: Rider and Co., 1953).

Leach, Abby. "The Ideal Curriculum for a Woman's College." *Publications of the Association of Collegiate Alumnae*, December 1898, pp. 17–21.

Lerner, Gerda, ed. *The Female Experience: An American Documentary* (Indianapolis: Bobbs-Merrill, 1977).

Lewis, Dio. *Talks about People's Stomachs* (Boston: Fields, Osgood and Co., 1870).

Lincoln, Mary. *Mrs. Lincoln's Boston Cook Book* (Boston: Roberts Brothers, 1883).

———. *The Peerless Cook Book* (Boston: Little, Brown, 1885).

———. *What to Have for Luncheon* (New York: Dodge, 1904).

McCollum, E. V. *The Newer Knowledge of Nutrition* (New York: Macmillan, 1918).

Macdonald, Elizabeth, and Forrester Macdonald. *Homemaking, a Profession for Men and Women* (Boston: Marshall Jones Co., 1927).

Mann, Mary Peabody. *Christianity in the Kitchen* (Boston: Ticknor and Fields, 1857).

Mark, Kenneth L. *Delayed by Fire* (Privately printed, 1945).

Massachusetts Bureau of Statistics of Labor. *Comparison of the Cost of Home-Made and Prepared Food* (Boston: Wright and Potter, 1901).

Melder, Keith. *Beginnings of Sisterhood* (New York: Schocken Books, 1977).

Milner, R. D., ed. *Dietary Studies in Boston and Springfield, Mass., Philadelphia, Pa., and Chicago, Ill.* (Washington, D.C.: Government Printing Office, 1903).

"Miss Farmer's School of Cookery. Announcement of Courses." Pamphlets, 1911–1912, 1912–1913.

"Miss Maria Parloa." *The Journal of Home Economics*, October 1909, pp. 378–85.

Mothers Club of Cambridge. Papers (manuscript, Schlesinger Library, Radcliffe College).

Mott, Frank Luther. *A History of American Magazines* (Cambridge, Mass.: Harvard University Press, 1938).

Nelson, Mariana T. "What Homemakers Learned About Purchasing Household Goods." *The Journal of Home Economics*, June 1932, pp. 519–20.

"The New York Cooking School." *Harper's New Monthly*, December 1879, pp. 22–9.

Nickerson, Jane. "Best-Seller—And Cooks' Friend." *The New York Times Magazine*, October 7, 1945, p. 16.

Owen, Catherine. *Progressive Housekeeping* (Boston: Houghton Mifflin, 1889).

———. *Ten Dollars Enough* (Boston: Houghton Mifflin, 1886).

Parker, Gail, ed. *The Oven Birds* (New York: Doubleday, 1972).

Parloa, Maria. *The Appledore Cookbook* (Boston: Graves and Ellis, 1872).

———. *Home Economics* (New York: The Century Co., 1906).

———. *Miss Parloa's Kitchen Companion* (Boston: Estes & Lauriat, 1887).

———. *Miss Parloa's New Cook Book and Marketing Guide* (Boston: Estes & Lauriat, 1880).

———. *Miss Parloa's Young Housekeeper* (Boston: Estes & Lauriat, 1894).

———. "The New England Kitchen." *The Century*, December 1891, pp. 315–17.

Pattison, Mary. *The Business of Home Management* (New York: Robert McBride, 1915).

"The People's Food—A Great National Inquiry." *The Review of Reviews*, June 1896, pp. 679–90.

Perkins, Dexter. *Yield of the Years* (Boston: Little, Brown, 1969).

Peyser, Ethel R. "A Quiet Factory Lunch Room." *The Journal of Home Economics*, December 1911, pp. 466–9.

Phelps, Elizabeth Stuart. *Beyond the Gates* (Boston: Houghton Mifflin, 1883).

———. *Chapters from a Life* (Boston: Houghton Mifflin, 1897).

———. *The Gates Ajar* (New York: The Regent Press, 1868).

———. *The Gates Between* (Boston: Houghton Mifflin, 1887).

———. *An Old Maid's Paradise* (Boston: Houghton Mifflin, 1885).

———. *The Silent Partner* (Boston: James R. Osgood, 1871).

———. *The Story of Avis* (Boston: James R. Osgood, 1877).

Plain Words about Food (Boston: Rockwell and Churchill Press, 1899).

Proceedings of the Lake Placid Conferences on Home Economics (New York: Lake Placid Club, 1901–1908).

Pryse, Marjorie, ed. *Selected Stories of Mary E. Wilkins Freeman* (New York: Norton, 1983).

Publications of the Association of Collegiate Alumnae. February 1908.

Ravenhill, Alice. *The Teaching of "Domestic Science" in the United States of America* (London: Wyman & Sons, Ltd, 1905).

Raymond, Edith. Papers (manuscript, Schlesinger Library, Radcliffe College).

Rhodes, Susie Root, and Grace Porter Hopkins, eds. *The Economic Administration Cook Book* (New York: Syndicate Publishing Co., 1913).

Richards, Ellen. *The Art of Right Living* (Boston: Whitcomb and Barrows, 1904).

———. *The Cost of Living* (New York: John Wiley and Sons, 1899).

———. *The Cost of Shelter* (New York: John Wiley and Sons, 1905).

———. *The Dietary Computer* (New York: John Wiley and Sons, 1902).

———. "Domestic Science." *The Outlook*, April 24, 1897, pp. 1078–80.

———. "Practical Suggestions for Applied Economics and Sociology in the College Curriculum." *Publications of the Association of Collegiate Alumnae*, January 1905, pp. 30–5.

———. "The Relation of College Women to Progress in Domestic Science." Paper presented to the Association of Collegiate Alumnae, October 24, 1890.

———. "Scientific Cooking-Studies in the New England Kitchen." *The Forum*, May 1893, pp. 355–61.

———. "The Social Significance of the Home Economics Movement." *The Journal of Home Economics*, April 1911, pp. 117–25.

Richards, Ellen, and S. Maria Elliott. *The Chemistry of Cooking and Cleaning* (Boston: Whitcomb and Barrows, 1916) (c. 1881).

Richmond, Mary. *Friendly Visiting Among the Poor* (New York: Macmillan, 1889).

Root, Waverley, and Richard de Rochemont. *Eating in America* (New York: William Morrow, 1976).

Rorer, Sarah Tyson. *Mrs. Rorer's New Cook Book* (Philadelphia: Arnold, 1902).

Rosenberg, Rosalind. *Beyond Separate Spheres* (New Haven: Yale University Press, 1982).

Rothman, Sheila M. *Woman's Proper Place* (New York: Basic Books, 1978).

Salmon, Lucy Maynard. *Domestic Service* (New York: Macmillan, 1897).

———. *Progress in the Household* (Boston: Houghton Mifflin, 1906).

School Lunches (Cincinnati: Procter & Gamble Co., 1926).

"The School of Housekeeping." Pamphlet, 1901–1902.

Sedgwick, Catharine Maria. *Home* (Boston: James Munroe, 1835).

———. *Married or Single?* (New York: Harper & Bros., 1857).

Sicherman, Barbara, and Carol Hurd Green, eds. *Notable American Women, The Modern Period* (Cambridge, Mass.: Harvard University Press, 1980).

Simmons, Amelia. *American Cookery* (Hartford, Conn.: Hudson and Goodwin, 1796).

Simmons College, *Annual Reports*, 1904.

The Simmons Review. Fall, 1952.

Sinclair, Upton. *The Jungle* (New York: Doubleday, Page and Co., 1906).

Sklar, Kathryn Kish. *Catharine Beecher* (New York: Norton, 1976).

Smedley, Emma, and R. D. Milner. *Dietary Studies in Public Institutions in Philadelphia, Pa.* (Washington, D.C.: Government Printing Office, 1910).

Smith, Mary Roberts. "Shall the College Curriculum Be Modified for Women?" *Publications of the Association of Collegiate Alumnae*, December 1898, pp. 1–15.

Smuts, Robert W. *Woman and Work in America* (New York: Schocken Books, 1971).

Stanton, Theodore, and Harriet Stanton Blatch, eds. *Elizabeth Cady Stanton* (New York: Harper and Bros., 1922).

Steele, Zulma. "Fannie Farmer and Her Cook Book," in Stein, Leon, ed., *Lives to Remember* (New York: Arno Press, 1974), pp. 66–71.

Stern, Jane and Michael. *Square Meals* (New York: Alfred A. Knopf, 1984).

Strasser, Susan. *Never Done* (New York: Pantheon, 1982).

Talbot, Marion. *More than Lore* (Chicago: University of Chicago Press, 1936).

———. *Publications of the Association of Collegiate Alumnae,* December 1898, pp. 25–8.

Tannahill, Reay. *Food in History* (London: Paladin, 1975).

Taylor, Mrs. Bayard. *Letters to a Young Housekeeper* (New York: Scribner's, 1892).

Teaching the Rudiments of Cooking in the Class Room (Washington, D.C.: Government Printing Office, 1906).

Training Schools of Cookery (Washington, D.C.: Government Printing Office, 1879).

True, Alfred Charles. *A History of Agricultural Education in the United States, 1785–1925* (Washington, D.C.: Government Printing Office, 1929).

Turgeon, Charlotte, and Nina Froud, eds. *Larousse Gastronomique* (New York: Crown, 1961).

Vegetable Cookery (Cincinnati: Procter & Gamble Co., 1926).

Wait, Charles. *Dietary Studies in Rural Regions* (Washington, D.C.: Government Printing Office, 1909).

Warner, Sam Bass. *Streetcar Suburbs* (Cambridge, Mass.: Harvard University Press, 1962).

Wasserman, Harvey. *Harvey Wasserman's History of the United States* (New York: Harper & Row, 1972).

Watson, Frank Dekker. *The Charity Organization Movement in the United States* (New York: Macmillan, 1922).

Weigley, Emma Seifrit. *Sarah Tyson Rorer* (Philadelphia: American Philosophical Society, 1977).

Welter, Barbara. *Dimity Convictions* (Athens: Ohio University Press, 1976).

Wentworth, Sarah E. "Some Experiments in Furnishing Lunches for School Children." Paper presented to the Association of Collegiate Alumnae, October 29, 1898.

West, Susan F. "The Education of Women for Leisure." *The Journal of Home Economics*, September 1927, pp. 491–550.

Willan, Anne. *Great Cooks and Their Recipes* (New York: McGraw-Hill, 1977.)

Williamson, Harold Francis. *Edward Atkinson* (Boston: Old Corner Book Store, 1934).

Winchell, Cora M. "Homemaking as a Phase of Citizenship." *The Journal of Home Economics*, January 1922, pp. 27–33.

Woman's Education Association. *Annual Reports*, 1872 ff. (Boston: Alfred Mudge and Son).

———. *Minutes of the Meetings, Boston Cooking School Committee*, February 15, 1872–December 5, 1882.

———. *Record of the Domestic Economy Committee*, 1903–4.

Woodhouse, Chase Going. *Business Opportunities for the Home Economist* (New York: McGraw-Hill, 1938).

Woods, Robert A., and Albert J. Kennedy. *Handbook of Settlements* (New York: Charities Publication Committee, 1911).

Woody, Thomas. *A History of Woman's Education in the United States* (New York: The Science Press, 1929).

Wright, Carroll D. *The Italians in Chicago* (Washington, D.C.: Government Printing Office, 1897).

Wright, Gwendolyn. *Moralism and the Model Home* (Chicago: University of Chicago Press, 1980).

Index